AF213820

Prostate Diseases - Management Strategies and Emerging Technologies

Edited by Ran Pang, Feiya Yang and Xianfeng Meng

Published in London, United Kingdom

Prostate Diseases - Management Strategies and Emerging Technologies
http://dx.doi.org/10.5772/intechopen.1003484
Edited by Ran Pang, Feiya Yang and Xianfeng Meng

Contributors
Ajay Bhandarkar, Anushavan Papoyan, Ditsapelo M. McFarland, Francesco Sessa, Ifiok Umana, Ildar Lutfarakhmanov, Jennifer Kimnuntluangi, Julius Akhaine, Luisa Moscardi, Marat Urmantsev, Meeta Singh, Necmi Bayraktar, Neha Pandey, Nisarg Mehta, Nita Khurana, Paolo Polverino, Peter Mironov, Ran Pang, Rishabh Handa, Sergio Contreras, Shaad Sarvar Vali, Shabnam Singh, Sophia Thomas, Tapan Jyoti Saikia, Vipul Ranjan Bhatt, William M. Baratedi

© The Editor(s) and the Author(s) 2025

The rights of the editor(s) and the author(s) have been asserted in accordance with the Copyright, Designs and Patents Act 1988. All rights to the book as a whole are reserved by INTECHOPEN LIMITED. The book as a whole (compilation) cannot be reproduced, distributed or used for commercial or non-commercial purposes without INTECHOPEN LIMITED's written permission. Enquiries concerning the use of the book should be directed to INTECHOPEN LIMITED rights and permissions department (permissions@intechopen.com).

Violations are liable to prosecution under the governing Copyright Law.

Individual chapters of this publication are distributed under the terms of the Creative Commons Attribution 4.0 License which permits commercial use, distribution and reproduction of the individual chapters, provided the original author(s) and source publication are appropriately acknowledged. If so indicated, certain images may not be included under the Creative Commons license. In such cases users will need to obtain permission from the license holder to reproduce the material. More details and guidelines concerning content reuse and adaptation can be found at http://www.intechopen.com/copyright-policy.html.

Notice

Statements and opinions expressed in the chapters are these of the individual contributors and not necessarily those of the editors or publisher. No responsibility is accepted for the accuracy of information contained in the published chapters. The publisher assumes no responsibility for any damage or injury to persons or property arising out of the use of any materials, instructions, methods or ideas contained in the book.

First published in London, United Kingdom, 2025 by IntechOpen
IntechOpen is the global imprint of INTECHOPEN LIMITED, registered in England and Wales, registration number: 11086078, 167-169 Great Portland Street, London, W1W 5PF, United Kingdom

For EU product safety concerns: IN TECH d.o.o., Prolaz Marije Krucifikse Kozulić 3, 51000 Rijeka, Croatia, info@intechopen.com or visit our website at intechopen.com.

British Library Cataloguing-in-Publication Data
A catalogue record for this book is available from the British Library

Prostate Diseases - Management Strategies and Emerging Technologies
Edited by Ran Pang, Feiya Yang and Xianfeng Meng
p. cm.
Print ISBN 978-0-85466-347-7
Online ISBN 978-0-85466-346-0
eBook (PDF) ISBN 978-0-85466-348-4

If disposing of this product, please recycle the paper responsibly.

We are IntechOpen, the world's leading publisher of Open Access books

Built by scientists, for scientists

7,400+
Open access books available

193,000+
International authors and editors

210M+
Downloads

156
Countries delivered to

Our authors are among the
Top 1%
most cited scientists

12.2%
Contributors from top 500 universities

WEB OF SCIENCE™

Selection of our books indexed in the Book Citation Index
in Web of Science™ Core Collection (BKCI)

Interested in publishing with us?
Contact book.department@intechopen.com

Numbers displayed above are based on latest data collected.
For more information visit www.intechopen.com

Meet the editors

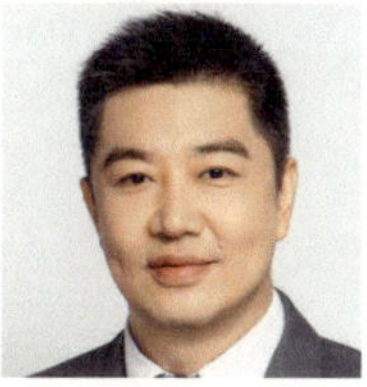

Ran Pang is a consultant urologist and a leader in functional urology and urodynamics at Guang'anmen Hospital, China Academy of Chinese Medical Sciences. After completing residency training, he was accepted to a clinical fellowship with Peking University. Subsequently, he joined a research fellowship at Mayo Clinic in the USA in 2011 and a urodynamic fellowship at Dalhousie University in Canada in 2015. As a leading expert, Prof. Pang serves on several international organizations and local professional committees. He is the chair of the Publication and Communication Committee, International Continence Society; vice chair of the Kidney Cancer Committee of Integrated Chinese and Western Medicine, China Anti-Cancer Association; and vice chair of the Female Urology Group of Urology Committee of Chinese Association of Integrative Medicine.

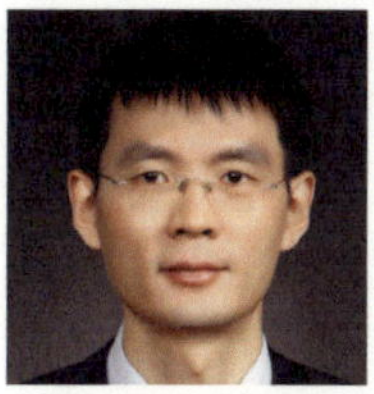

Feiya Yang is a consultant urologist and an associate professor in the Department of Urology at the National Cancer Center / National Clinical Research Center for Cancer / Cancer Hospital at the Chinese Academy of Medical Sciences and Peking Union Medical College. As a leading expert in urological oncology, Dr. Yang also serves on several national as well as local professional committees, such as the standing committee member of the Kidney Cancer Committee of Integrated Chinese and Western Medicine, China Anti-Cancer Association and the general secretary of Urological Oncology Committee and Beijing Oncology Association. He has also won eight professional awards, including the first prize in the scientific and technological progress of integrated traditional Chinese and Western medicine in 2020.

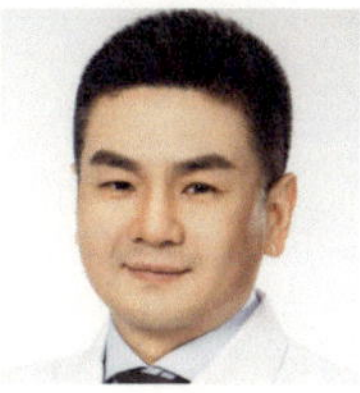

Xianfeng Meng is a consultant urologist and an associate professor at the Department of Urology, an affiliated hospital of Changchun University of Traditional Chinese Medicine. As a leading expert, Dr. Meng also serves on several national as well as local professional committees, such as the chair of the Kidney Cancer Committee of Integrated Chinese and Western Medicine, China Anti-Cancer Association; Vice Chair of the Men's Specialist Committee of the Jilin Association of Integrative Medicine; and the standing member of the Urology Committee, Jilin Medical Association.

Contents

Preface

The prostate, as an organ unique to men, can produce fluids that feed and protect sperm. Once the prostate has any problems, the patient may experience lower urinary tract symptoms (LUTS) and painful ejaculation because, anatomically, the prostate surrounds the proximal urethra and two ejaculatory ducts. Benign prostatic hyperplasia (BPH), prostate cancer (PCa), and prostatitis are generally the most common conditions affecting the prostate.

Besides providing an overview of the latest developments in the management of prostate diseases, section 1 of the book demonstrates the histopathological evaluation of different prostate diseases. The more histopathological characteristics of prostate disorders are understood, the more precise management strategy can be developed.

BPH is the primary cause of bladder outlet obstruction, which results in LUTS significantly in ageing men. Surgery is an effective approach to relieve obstruction. Traditionally, transurethral resection of the prostate (TURP) has been considered the gold standard of procedure for BPH/LUTS. Recently, the significant success of anatomical endoscopic enucleation of the prostate with various energy instruments has led to its widespread usage in clinical practice. Prostate enucleation using a holmium laser (HoLEP) is the most popular procedure. Moreover, minimally invasive surgical procedures, such as transperineal laser ablation of the prostate, have also been used for certain specific populations due to the minimal impact on male sexual function. In addition to the impact on sexual function, the relationship between BPH and male infertility has also attracted widespread attention. The contents in section 2 of the book discuss the effects of BPH and its related treatment on male infertility aside from introducing new surgical approaches.

PCa is the second most common cancer in the male population. With several novel drugs being launched, the treatment strategies for PCa have evolved in the past years. Not only are the different management strategies and surgical approaches discussed, but the issue of PCa management in the poor region of Africa is also analyzed in section 3 of the book.

As most readers would expect, experts and researchers from different countries present the latest advances and innovations in the field of prostate diseases. The contents of this book provide readers with crucial, up-to-date information, although they cannot cover every aspect of prostate diseases.

Ran Pang
Department of Urology,
Guang'anmen Hospital,
China Academy of Chinese Medical Sciences,
Beijing, China

Feiya Yang
Department of Urology,
National Cancer Center/National Clinical Research Center for Cancer/
Cancer Hospital,
Chinese Academy of Medical Sciences and Peking Union Medical College,
Beijing, China

Xianfeng Meng
Department of Urology,
Affiliated Hospital of Changchun University of Traditional Chinese Medicine,
Changchun, China

Section 1

Introduction and Basic Concepts

Chapter 1

Introductory Chapter: Innovations and Emerging Strategies in Prostate Diseases Management

Ran Pang

1. Introduction

The prostate gland, a crucial component of the male reproductive system, plays a pivotal role in the production and delivery of semen. Located just below the bladder and in front of the rectum, it surrounds the proximal urethra and two ejaculatory ducts. Therefore, the patient may experience ejaculatory or urination-related symptoms once any prostate issues have developed. The primary function of the prostate gland is to secrete an alkaline fluid, a significant portion of semen, which contributes to sperm protection in the vagina's acidic environment. Not only can the prostatic fluid balance the vagina's acidity, but it also contains the supportive proteins and enzymes that may nourish sperm and extend their lifespan. Additionally, the muscle tissue in the prostate gland contracts during ejaculation to aid in the expulsion of semen from the body. Initially, the prostate is anatomically considered to be composed of five lobes: the anterior, median, posterior, and two lateral lobes. Later, McNeal developed a zonal anatomy model of the prostate based on clinical and histological features, which divided the prostate into glandular and non-glandular components [1]. The former includes three zones: transition zone (TZ), central zone (CZ), and peripheral zone (PZ), whereas the latter is named as anterior fibromuscular stroma (AFMS). Evidence has demonstrated that distinct prostate zones differ significantly in terms of histological and pathogenetic features, embryonic origin, malignant propensity, and androgen expression [2].

It seems to be inevitable for men to be bothered by various prostate diseases in their lifetime. In general, the most common conditions affecting the prostate are prostatitis, benign prostatic hyperplasia (BPH), and prostate cancer (PCa). Of those, BPH is more likely to develop in the TZ, while PCa and prostatitis are more likely to occur in the PZ [2]. As the awareness of these conditions continues to grow, many new management techniques and therapy modalities are emerging.

2. Prostatitis

Prostatitis is one of the most common urology disorders in men younger than 50 years and significantly weakens patients' quality of life (QoL). The reported prevalence ranged from 8.5% to 16%, depending on the method used to investigate [3, 4]. To standardize the diagnosis of prostatitis, the National Institutes of Health

(NIH) developed a classification, in which prostatitis is categorized into four types based on patients' clinical manifestations as well as the white blood cells and bacteria identified in expressed prostatic secretions (EPS) (**Table 1**) [5].

In terms of the management of prostatitis, culture-guided antibiotic treatment is the standard strategy for acute (type I) and chronic bacterial prostatitis (type II) because bacterial infection is considered the etiology of the two types of prostatitis. On the other hand, it remains a challenge to manage chronic prostatitis/chronic pelvic pain syndrome (CP/CPPS) (type III) since its exact cause is still not fully understood. Actually, the treatment approaches of CP/CPPS have been mainly focused on symptom management. Recently, the UPOINTS system, developed to categorize diverse symptoms of CP/CPPS, provides insight into symptom-directed treatment. According to the algorithm, the symptoms of CP/CPPS are classified into seven domains: urinary symptoms (U), psychosocial disorders (P), organ-specific symptoms (O), infection (I), neurologic symptoms (N), tenderness (T), and sexual dysfunction (S) [6].

Regarding urinary symptoms, alpha-blockers are the most commonly used medication in clinical practice. A network meta-analysis demonstrated that alpha-blocker monotherapy or in combination with antibiotics could considerably relieve the voiding symptoms as well as the pain when compared to placebo [7]. The results from a Cochrane systematic review also showed that short-term alpha-blocker therapy could lower the patients' National Institutes of Health Chronic Prostatitis Symptom Index (NIH-CPSI) total scores as well as the sub-scores of urinary symptoms, pain, and QoL compared to placebo [8]. Unfortunately, the quality of the evidence is very low due to the high risk of bias, inconsistency, and imprecision in most studies.

The relationship between CP/CPPS and psychosocial disorder has been reported [9]. The selective 5-serotonin and norepinephrine reuptake inhibitor, as a kind of antidepressant, is also used to manage psychosocial symptoms in patients with CP/CPPS. A prospective, open-labeled study showed that duloxetine combined with doxazosin could reduce the NIH-CPSI and short-form McGill Pain questionnaire (SF-MPQ) scores more significantly than doxazosin alone and in combination with sertraline [10].

In terms of organ-specific symptoms, such as specific prostate tenderness and hematospermia, some phytomedicines including quercetin, pollen extract, and eviprostat have been reported to be effective [11–13].

Type	Description	WBC in EPS	Bacteria in EPS
I	Acute bacterial prostatitis (ABP)	+*	+*
II	Chronic bacterial prostatitis (CBP)	+	+
III	Chronic prostatitis/chronic pelvic pain syndrome (CP/CPPS)		
IIIa	Inflammatory	+	–
IIIb	Non-inflammatory	–	–
IV	Asymptomatic inflammatory prostatitis (AIP)	+	–

**Prostate massage is not recommended because of the bacterial dissemination risk. WBC: white blood cells; EPS: expressed prostatic secretions.*

Table 1.
NIH classification of prostatitis.

Antimicrobial treatment is the most widely used approach to infection. A randomized controlled trial (RCT) showed that levofloxacin alone or added on to terazosin presents a higher response rate as well as a more significant decrease in white blood cells (WBC) in expressed prostatic secretions (EPS) in comparison with terazosin monotherapy [14]. However, another RCT revealed that levofloxacin failed to present a better efficacy in managing CP/CPPS when compared to placebo [15]. The exact role of antimicrobial treatment in patients with CP/CPPS needs to be further confirmed in well-designed RCTs.

Although analgesics have been considered the common medication for the management of neurological symptoms in patients with CP/CPPS, a RCT found no significant difference in the percentage of responders who achieved a 6-point decrease in NIH-CPSI total score between 6-week pregabalin therapy and placebo [16]. By contrast, a number of studies present the effectiveness of botulinum neurotoxin type-A (BoNT-A) in the treatment of CP/CPPS. The results from an RCT showed that transurethral intraprostatic BoNT-A injection could relieve pain and improve QoL more effectively compared to placebo [17]. Similarly, another RCT found transurethral intraprostatic BoNT-A injection resulted in a significant reduction in NIH-CPSI and visual analog scale (VAS) scores while not in the control group (no treatment) [18]. In terms of different injection approaches, it is reported that the transrectal route was associated with a more significant improvement compared to the transurethral route [19]. Besides conventional treatment, growing evidence showed that acupuncture played a superior role in the management of CP/CPPS. The finding from two recent meta-analyses demonstrated that acupuncture had larger effect sizes in reducing NIH-CPSI total score as well as the sub-scores of each domain compared to sham acupuncture and modern medicine [20, 21]. Another meta-analysis concluded that the optional acupoints might focus on the combination of acupoints from CV3, CV4, BL32, SP6, and SP9 after investigating different acupoint selection strategies [22].

The spasm and/or trigger points in the pelvic floor muscles may be identified during examination in the patients presenting tenderness. The pelvic floor physical therapy is generally used as the first-line treatment for these patients. It is reported that both transrectal microwave thermotherapy and transrectal radiofrequency hyperthermia can improve the NIH-CPSI score in patients with CP/CPPS [23, 24]. The results from a phase II clinical trial showed that transurethral needle ablation was effective in relieving the symptoms of CP/CPPS, although the approach was initially used to treat BPH [25]. In addition, increasing amounts of evidence support the effectiveness of extracorporeal shock wave therapy (ESWT) in treating prostatitis. An RCT showed a significant improvement in CP/CPPS symptoms and QoL in the ESWT group while not in the sham therapy group during the 12-week follow-up period [26]. Some studies further presented the long-term efficacy of ESWT. Findings from these studies revealed that patients' NIH-CPSI score as well as the international index of erectile function (IIEF) were significantly improved as early as the 2nd week to the 12th week and remained stabilized by the 12-month follow-up [27, 28]. Two recent meta-analyses demonstrated that ESWT could more significantly improve the NIH-CPSI total score and the sub-scores of each domain compared to sham intervention [29, 30].

Type 5 Phosphodiesterase (PDE-5) inhibitors are the common medication for the treatment of erectile dysfunction. It is revealed that PDE-5 is expressed not only in PZ and TZ but in AFMS of the prostate gland [31]. The PDE-5 inhibitors can be used to treat CP/CPPS due to their reported role in the suppression of inflammation. The findings from an RCT showed that Tadalafil could improve the NIH-CPSI total score, the urinary score, and the QoL more significantly than placebo [32]. The potential mechanism may be associated with its role in relaxing prostatic smooth muscle and reducing prostatic reflux of urine [33].

3. BPH

BPH, characterized by overgrowth of the epithelium and stroma of prostate gland histologically, is a common condition in elderly men. Bladder outlet obstruction caused by the enlarged prostate is the primary cause of lower urinary tract symptoms (LUTS) in aging male population. The prevalence of both LUTS and BPH significantly rises with age, affecting over 80% of men by the age of 70 [34]. Historically, surgery was the best way to alleviate the LUTS caused by benign prostatic obstruction (BPO). However, the management strategy has been markedly changed with the launch of numerous new medications over the past decades. Nowadays, there are six pharmacological classes available for the treatment of LUTS due to BPO, either alone or in combination. These medications include alpha-blockers, 5-alpha reductase inhibitors, PDE-5 inhibitors, anticholinergics, beta-3 agonists, and phytotherapy.

Compared with monotherapy, combination therapy may be associated with more significant efficacy. Several RCTs have provided substantial evidence of the efficacy of alpha-blockers combined with 5-alpha reductase inhibitors in the management of BPH/LUTS. Of those, MTOPS and CombAT studies showed long-term efficacy. Combination therapy was significantly superior to monotherapy not only in improving the LUTS and maximum urine flow rate (Qmax) but also in lowering the risk of clinical progression during a 4-year follow-up period [35, 36]. For patients with coexisted voiding and storage LUTS, alpha-blockers combined with anticholinergics or beta-3 agonists are the common treatment strategies. According to the findings from a Cochrane systematic review, combination therapy with alpha-blockers and anticholinergics only had a small effect size in improving the international prostate symptom score (IPSS) and QoL, when compared with alpha-blocker monotherapy [37]. The results from a meta-analysis showed that alpha-blockers combined with beta-3 agonists might be more effective in reducing the mean number of micturitions per day, the urgency episodes per day, and overactive bladder (OAB) symptom score compared to alpha-blockers combined with placebo [38]. Another Cochrane systematic review demonstrated that combination therapy with alpha-blockers and PDE-5 inhibitors had a greater improvement in IPSS, Qmax, as well as the international index of erectile function (IIEF-5) score in comparison with alpha-blockers alone [39]. In addition, a network meta-analysis involving 55 RCTs showed that combination of PDE-5 inhibitors and α-blockers could be the optimal strategy that improved IPSS more significantly not only than monotherapy but also than any other combination strategies [40].

Surgery is believed to be a therapeutic option for the patients who fail to respond to pharmacological therapy, experience clinically intolerable adverse drug reactions, or present complications. Traditionally, transurethral resection of the prostate (TURP) has been considered the gold standard of procedure for BPH/LUTS. Recently, anatomical endoscopic enucleation of the prostate with different energy equipment has been widely used in clinical practice due to its notable effectiveness. Holmium laser enucleation of the prostate (HoLEP) is the most common procedure. A meta-analysis found that HoLEP exhibited a greater curative efficacy and fewer adverse events at 6, 12, and 24 months following surgery when compared to TURP [41].

Moreover, a number of minimally invasive surgical procedures have also emerged due to the development of novel technologies in recent years. These procedures actually have some advantages, such as being performed under local anesthesia, quicker recovery, fewer complications compared to TURP. On the other hand, these minimally invasive therapies might be associated with a higher failure rate and less symptom improvement [42]. These procedures mainly include prostatic urethral lift, prostatic artery embolization (PAE), aquablation, and water vapor therapy.

4. PCa

PCa is the fourth most common cancer worldwide and the second most prevalent malignancy in male population. In general, about 80% of newly diagnosed PCa patients are localized, whereas 20% are metastatic or advanced. When making a treatment strategy, the patients' stage of PCa, risk factors, comorbidity, and preference all need to be taken into consideration.

4.1 Localized and locally advanced PCa

The treatment strategy for localized PCa is normally developed depending on the risk of clinical progression. The progression risk of PCa is generally categorized using International Society for Urological Pathology (ISUP) grading, with ISUP grade groups 1–2 being low risk and ISUP grade groups 3–5 being intermediate to high risk [43]. Another widely accepted risk stratification of PCa is D'Amico classification system, in which the patients are classified into low, intermediate, or high-risk groups based on PSA, Gleason score, and clinical tumor (cT) stage [44]. Although laparoscopic or robot-assisted radical prostatectomy remains a golden standard for localized PCa with intermediate to high risk, radiotherapy is increasingly used with the development of image-guided techniques. The image-guided radiotherapy provides better cancer control because precise irradiation allows delivering high-beam doses while reducing toxicities to surrounding organs [45]. Regarding low-risk localized PCa, active surveillance is a common therapeutic option with clear benefits for QoL. In terms of locally advanced PCa, androgen deprivation therapies (ADT) in conjunction with either radical prostatectomy or radiotherapy can result in a better prognosis [46].

4.2 Metastatic hormone-sensitive prostate cancer (mHSPC)

In order to estimate the prognosis of mHSPC, several studies developed some criteria to stratify the patients. In the CHAARTED study, patients with mHSPC were divided into high-volume and low-volume groups based on metastatic burden. The former was defined as the occurrence of visceral metastases and/or at least four bone metastases, with at least one lesion outside the pelvis and vertebral bodies, while the latter referred to others [47]. LATITUDE study grouped patients into high-risk and low-risk poor prognosis. Once the patients had two or more high-risk factors, including at least three bone metastases, visceral metastases, and ISUP 4–5, they were defined as high-risk; otherwise, they were considered as low-risk [48]. Generally, patients with high-volume diseases or high-risk poor prognosis need more intensive treatments.

ADT is believed to be a cornerstone of treatment for mHSPC since PCa was identified as an androgen-sensitive disease by Huggins and Hodges about 80 years ago. However, accumulated evidence suggests that ADT alone is insufficient to offer long-term survival and sustained disease control, especially for high-volume or high-risk mHSPC. In recent years, several combination therapy strategies have emerged to manage mHSPC. According to the findings from the STAMPEDE trial, ADT combined with docetaxel presented a significant benefit on overall survival (OS) compared to ADT alone [49]. The CHAARTED trial showed that combination therapy with ADT and docetaxel had a superior OS in patients with high-volume PCa, while not in those with low-volume PCa, when compared to ADT alone [50]. Some studies assessed the role of combination of ADT and androgen receptor signaling inhibitors (ARSI) in management of mHSPC. The LATITUDE study showed that ADT combined with abiraterone acetate and prednisone (AAP) was significantly superior to ADT monotherapy in OS [48]. Based on the results of TITAN study, the combination of ADT and apalutamide had a significant survival benefit over ADT combined with placebo [51]. In addition, two trials further investigated the effectiveness of triple combination therapy (ADT+ ARSI+ docetaxel) in treating mHSPC. The ARASENS study showed that ADT combined with darolutamide and docetaxel reduced the risk of death by 25% in comparison with the combination of ADT and docetaxel [52]. The PEACE-1 trial showed similar results in triple combination therapy with ADT, AAP, and docetaxel [53].

4.3 Castration-resistant prostate cancer (CRPC)

Despite responding to initial ADT, most patients will inevitably progress to CRPC within 2–3 years. Some patients may experience non-metastatic CRPC (nmCRPC), which is characterized as a persistently elevated PSA in spite of castration levels of testosterone and no conventional radiographic evidence of metastasis, before the metastasis occurs. Recently, a perspective has emerged suggesting that patients with nmCRPC actually have small metastatic lesions that failed to be detected by conventional imaging. Nowadays, ARSI including apalutamide, enzalutamide, and darolutamide have been the standard management for nmCRPC due to their notable benefits on metastasis-free survival [54].

In terms of metastatic CRPC (mCRPC), the first-line treatment varies from individual to individual. An early study showed that docetaxel was associated with a better OS (17.5 vs. 15.6 months) and radiographic progression-free survival (rPFS) (6.3 vs. 3.2 months) compared to mitoxantrone [55]. According to the COU-AA-302 trial, AAP was superior to placebo in both OS (34.7 vs. 30.3 months) and rPFS (16.5 vs. 8.3 months) in chemotherapy-naïve mCRPC patients [56]. The PREVAIL study presented similar results. The OS and rPFS in the enzalutamide group were significantly longer than in placebo group [57].

For mCRPC patients failing to respond to docetaxel, ARSI are still a treatment option. The COU-AA-301 study showed the superiority of AAP in OS (15.8 vs. 11.2 months) and rPFS (5.6 vs. 3.6 months) in patients with docetaxel-resistant mCRPC [58]. Similar results were found in AFFIRM trial. The OS and rPFS in enzalutamide group were 18.4 and 8.3 months, respectively, which were significantly longer than in placebo group (13.6 and 2.9 months) [59]. Besides ARSI, cabazitaxel, as a novel taxane, has been reported to be effective for docetaxel-resistant mCRPC. The CARD study presented that cabazitaxel led to a longer OS compared to AAP or enzalutamide [60]. Additionally, Radium 223 can be an optional treatment for patients with multiple symptomatic bone metastases and no visceral metastases. Based on the findings from ALSYMPCA study, Radium 223 not only relieved the metastatic bone pain significantly but also was associated with a better OS when compared with placebo [61]. For patients with mutations in DNA damage repair genes, poly (ADP-ribose) polymerase (PARP) inhibitors can lead to PCa cell death and consequently improve patients' outcomes. The PROfound study demonstrated that Olaparib achieved a superior OS and rPFS compared to AAP or enzalutamide in patients with BRCA1, BRCA2, or ATM mutation [62]. A recent meta-analysis suggested that the combination of PARP inhibitors and ARSI reduced the risk of death by 16% [63].

5. Summary and perspective

With several novel drugs and techniques emerging, the treatment strategies for prostate diseases have rapidly evolved in the past years. The book aims to provide cutting-edge thinking and innovative techniques in the management of prostate diseases. Not only is the latest evidence demonstrated but also the state-of-the-art treatment concepts and insights from the leading experts are also showcased. The volume caters to a diverse reader. It offers clinicians precise treatment strategies, equips patients with essential background knowledge for communicating with doctors, and provides researchers with valuable research insights. Additionally, this book could serve as a catalyst. If it sparks thought in its readers, a more promising future lies ahead for patients with prostate diseases.

Author details

Ran Pang
Guang'anmen Hospital, China Academy of Chinese Medical Sciences, Beijing, China

*Address all correspondence to: pangran2002@gmail.com

IntechOpen

© 2025 The Author(s). Licensee IntechOpen. This chapter is distributed under the terms of the Creative Commons Attribution License (http://creativecommons.org/licenses/by/4.0), which permits unrestricted use, distribution, and reproduction in any medium, provided the original work is properly cited. (cc) BY

References

[1] McNeal JE. The zonal anatomy of the prostate. The Prostate. 1981;**2**(1):35-49

[2] Yu XD, Yan SS, Liu RJ, Zhang YS. Apparent differences in prostate zones: Susceptibility to prostate cancer, benign prostatic hyperplasia and prostatitis. International Urology and Nephrology. 2024;**56**(8):2451-2458

[3] Collins MM, Meigs JB, Barry MJ, Walker Corkery E, Giovannucci E, Kawachi I. Prevalence and correlates of prostatitis in the health professionals follow-up study cohort. The Journal of Urology. 2002;**167**(3):1363-1366

[4] Nickel JC, Downey J, Hunter D, Clark J. Prevalence of prostatitis-like symptoms in a population based study using the National Institutes of Health chronic prostatitis symptom index. The Journal of Urology. 2001;**165**(3):842-845

[5] Krieger JN, Nyberg L Jr, Nickel JC. NIH consensus definition and classification of prostatitis. Journal of the American Medical Association. 1999;**282**(3):236-237

[6] Magri V, Marras E, Restelli A, Wagenlehner FM, Perletti G. Multimodal therapy for category III chronic prostatitis/chronic pelvic pain syndrome in UPOINTS phenotyped patients. Experimental and Therapeutic Medicine. 2015;**9**(3):658-666

[7] Anothaisintawee T, Attia J, Nickel JC, Thammakraisorn S, Numthavaj P, McEvoy M, et al. Management of chronic prostatitis/chronic pelvic pain syndrome: A systematic review and network meta-analysis. Journal of the American Medical Association. 2011;**305**(1):78-86

[8] Franco JV, Turk T, Jung JH, Xiao YT, Iakhno S, Tirapegui FI, et al. Pharmacological interventions for treating chronic prostatitis/chronic pelvic pain syndrome. The Cochrane Database of Systematic Reviews. 2019;**10**(10):Cd012552

[9] Riegel B, Bruenahl CA, Ahyai S, Bingel U, Fisch M, Löwe B. Assessing psychological factors, social aspects and psychiatric co-morbidity associated with Chronic Prostatitis/Chronic Pelvic Pain Syndrome (CP/CPPS) in men—A systematic review. Journal of Psychosomatic Research. 2014;**77**(5):333-350

[10] Zhang M, Li H, Ji Z, Dong D, Yan S. Clinical study of duloxetine hydrochloride combined with doxazosin for the treatment of pain disorder in chronic prostatitis/chronic pelvic pain syndrome: An observational study. Medicine. 2017;**96**(10):e6243

[11] Iwamura H, Koie T, Soma O, Matsumoto T, Imai A, Hatakeyama S, et al. Eviprostat has an identical effect compared to pollen extract (Cernilton) in patients with chronic prostatitis/chronic pelvic pain syndrome: A randomized, prospective study. BMC Urology. 2015;**15**:120

[12] Shoskes DA, Zeitlin SI, Shahed A, Rajfer J. Quercetin in men with category III chronic prostatitis: A preliminary prospective, double-blind, placebo-controlled trial. Urology. 1999;**54**(6):960-963

[13] Wagenlehner FM, Schneider H, Ludwig M, Schnitker J, Brähler E, Weidner W. A pollen extract (Cernilton) in patients with inflammatory chronic prostatitis-chronic pelvic pain syndrome:

A multicentre, randomised, prospective, double-blind, placebo-controlled phase 3 study. European Urology. 2009;**56**(3):544-551

[14] Wang J, Yan D, Liang K, Xu Z. A randomized controlled trial of levofloxacin, terazosin, and combination therapy in patients with category III chronic prostatitis/chronic pelvic pain syndrome. International Urology and Nephrology. 2016;**48**(1):13-18

[15] Nickel JC, Downey J, Clark J, Casey RW, Pommerville PJ, Barkin J, et al. Levofloxacin for chronic prostatitis/chronic pelvic pain syndrome in men: A randomized placebo-controlled multicenter trial. Urology. 2003;**62**(4):614-617

[16] Pontari MA, Krieger JN, Litwin MS, White PC, Anderson RU, McNaughton-Collins M, et al. Pregabalin for the treatment of men with chronic prostatitis/chronic pelvic pain syndrome: A randomized controlled trial. Archives of Internal Medicine. 2010;**170**(17):1586-1593

[17] Falahatkar S, Shahab E, Gholamjani Moghaddam K, Kazemnezhad E. Transurethral intraprostatic injection of botulinum neurotoxin type A for the treatment of chronic prostatitis/chronic pelvic pain syndrome: Results of a prospective pilot double-blind and randomized placebo-controlled study. BJU International. 2015;**116**(4):641-649

[18] Abdel-Meguid TA, Mosli HA, Farsi H, Alsayyad A, Tayib A, Sait M, et al. Treatment of refractory category III nonbacterial chronic prostatitis/chronic pelvic pain syndrome with intraprostatic injection of onabotulinumtoxinA: A prospective controlled study. The Canadian Journal of Urology. 2018;**25**(2):9273-9280

[19] El-Enen MA, Abou-Farha M, El-Abd A, El-Tatawy H, Tawfik A, El-Abd S, et al. Intraprostatic injection of botulinum toxin-A in patients with refractory chronic pelvic pain syndrome: The transurethral vs. transrectal approach. Arab Journal of Urology. 2015;**13**(2):94-99

[20] Pan J, Jin S, Xie Q, Wang Y, Wu Z, Sun J, et al. Acupuncture for chronic prostatitis or chronic pelvic pain syndrome: An updated systematic review and meta-analysis. Pain Research and Management. 2023;**2023**:7754876

[21] Qin Z, Guo J, Chen H, Wu J. Acupuncture for chronic prostatitis/chronic pelvic pain syndrome: A GRADE-assessed systematic review and meta-analysis. European Urology Open Science. 2022;**46**:55-67

[22] Zhang W, Fang Y, Shi M, Zhang M, Chen Y, Zhou T. Optimal acupoint and session of acupuncture for patients with chronic prostatitis/chronic pelvic pain syndrome: A meta-analysis. Translational Andrology and Urology. 2021;**10**(1):143-153

[23] Gao M, Ding H, Zhong G, Lu J, Wang H, Li Q, et al. The effects of transrectal radiofrequency hyperthermia on patients with chronic prostatitis and the changes of MDA, NO, SOD, and Zn levels in pretreatment and posttreatment. Urology. 2012;**79**(2):391-396

[24] Jin J-X, Wang H-Z, Zhai Z-X, Ma B-L, Li Q-F, Xiao N, et al. Transrectal microwave thermotherapy causing a short-time influence on sperm quality in Chinese chronic nonbacterial prostatitis patients. Asian Journal of Andrology. 2017;**19**(5):548-553

[25] Chiang PH, Chiang CP. Therapeutic effect of transurethral needle ablation in non-bacterial prostatitis: Chronic pelvic

pain syndrome type IIIa. International Journal of Urology : Official Journal of the Japanese Urological Association. 2004;**11**(2):97-102

[26] Zimmermann R, Cumpanas A, Miclea F, Janetschek G. Extracorporeal shock wave therapy for the treatment of chronic pelvic pain syndrome in males: A randomised, double-blind, placebo-controlled study. European Urology. 2009;**56**(3):418-424

[27] Al Edwan GM, Muheilan MM, Atta ON. Long term efficacy of extracorporeal shock wave therapy [ESWT] for treatment of refractory chronic abacterial prostatitis. Annals of Medicine and Surgery. 2012;**2017**(14):12-17

[28] Skaudickas D, Lenčiauskas P, Skaudickas A, Undžytė G. Low intensity extracorporeal shockwave therapy for chronic pelvic pain syndrome: Long-term follow-up. Open Medicine (Warsaw, Poland). 2023;**18**(1):20230832

[29] Li G, Man L. Low-intensity extracorporeal shock wave therapy for male chronic pelvic pain syndrome: A systematic review and meta-analysis. Translational Andrology and Urology. 2021;**10**(3):1202-1211

[30] Mykoniatis I, Pyrgidis N, Sokolakis I, Sountoulides P, Hatzichristodoulou G, Apostolidis A, et al. Low-intensity shockwave therapy for the management of chronic prostatitis/chronic pelvic pain syndrome: A systematic review and meta-analysis. BJU International. 2021;**128**(2):144-152

[31] Iwata T, Fujihara A, Shiraishi T, Yamada Y, Hongo F, Ukimura O. Higher expression of phosphodiesterase type 5 in the anterior fibromuscular stroma of the human prostate. World Journal of Urology. 2020;**38**(11):2915-2921

[32] Tawfik AM, Radwan MH, Abdulmonem M, Abo-Elenen M, Elgamal SA, Aboufarha MO. Tadalafil monotherapy in management of chronic prostatitis/chronic pelvic pain syndrome: A randomized double-blind placebo controlled clinical trial. World Journal of Urology. 2022;**40**(10):2505-2511

[33] Grimsley SJ, Khan MH, Jones GE. Mechanism of phosphodiesterase 5 inhibitor relief of prostatitis symptoms. Medical Hypotheses. 2007;**69**(1):25-26

[34] Egan KB. The epidemiology of benign prostatic hyperplasia associated with lower urinary tract symptoms: Prevalence and incident rates. Urologic Clinics of North America. 2016;**43**(3):289-297

[35] McConnell JD, Roehrborn CG, Bautista OM, Andriole GL Jr, Dixon CM, Kusek JW, et al. The long-term effect of doxazosin, finasteride, and combination therapy on the clinical progression of benign prostatic hyperplasia. The New England Journal of Medicine. 2003;**349**(25):2387-2398

[36] Roehrborn CG, Siami P, Barkin J, Damião R, Major-Walker K, Nandy I, et al. The effects of combination therapy with dutasteride and tamsulosin on clinical outcomes in men with symptomatic benign prostatic hyperplasia: 4-year results from the CombAT study. European Urology. 2010;**57**(1):123-131

[37] Pang R, Zhou XY, Wang X, Wang B, Yin XL, Bo H, et al. Anticholinergics combined with alpha-blockers for treating lower urinary tract symptoms related to benign prostatic obstruction. The Cochrane Database of Systematic Reviews. 2021;**2**(2):Cd012336

[38] Su S, Lin J, Liang L, Liu L, Chen Z, Gao Y. The efficacy and safety

of mirabegron on overactive bladder induced by benign prostatic hyperplasia in men receiving tamsulosin therapy: A systematic review and meta-analysis. Medicine. 2020;**99**(4):e18802

[39] Pattanaik S, Mavuduru RS, Panda A, Mathew JL, Agarwal MM, Hwang EC, et al. Phosphodiesterase inhibitors for lower urinary tract symptoms consistent with benign prostatic hyperplasia. The Cochrane Database of Systematic Reviews. 2018;**11**(11):Cd010060

[40] Fan Z, Shi H, Zhang J, Wang H, Wang J. Comparative efficacy of different drugs for lower urinary tract symptoms due to benign prostatic hyperplasia: A Bayesian network meta-analysis. Frontiers in Pharmacology. 2022;**13**:763184

[41] Chen F, Chen Y, Zou Y, Wang Y, Wu X, Chen M. Comparison of holmium laser enucleation and transurethral resection of prostate in benign prostatic hyperplasia: A systematic review and meta-analysis. Journal of International Medical Research. 2023;**51**(8):3000605231190763

[42] Christidis D, McGrath S, Perera M, Manning T, Bolton D, Lawrentschuk N. Minimally invasive surgical therapies for benign prostatic hypertrophy: The rise in minimally invasive surgical therapies. Prostate International. 2017;**5**(2):41-46

[43] Epstein JI, Egevad L, Amin MB, Delahunt B, Srigley JR, Humphrey PA. The 2014 International Society of Urological Pathology (ISUP) consensus conference on Gleason grading of prostatic carcinoma: Definition of grading patterns and proposal for a new grading system. The American Journal of Surgical Pathology. 2016;**40**(2):244-252

[44] Hernandez DJ, Nielsen ME, Han M, Partin AW. Contemporary evaluation of the D'amico risk classification of prostate cancer. Urology. 2007;**70**(5):931-935

[45] Wang S, Tang W, Luo H, Jin F, Wang Y. The role of image-guided radiotherapy in prostate cancer: A systematic review and meta-analysis. Clinical and Translational Radiation Oncology. 2023;**38**:81-89

[46] Amiya Y, Yamada Y, Sugiura M, Sasaki M, Shima T, Suzuki N, et al. Treatment of locally advanced prostate cancer (stage T3). Japanese Journal of Clinical Oncology. 2017;**47**(3):257-261

[47] Gravis G, Boher JM, Chen YH, Liu G, Fizazi K, Carducci MA, et al. Burden of metastatic castrate naive prostate cancer patients, to identify men more likely to benefit from early docetaxel: Further analyses of CHAARTED and GETUG-AFU15 studies. European Urology. 2018;**73**(6):847-855

[48] Fizazi K, Tran N, Fein L, Matsubara N, Rodriguez-Antolin A, Alekseev BY, et al. Abiraterone plus prednisone in metastatic, castration-sensitive prostate cancer. The New England Journal of Medicine. 2017;**377**(4):352-360

[49] Clarke NW, Ali A, Ingleby FC, Hoyle A, Amos CL, Attard G, et al. Addition of docetaxel to hormonal therapy in low- and high-burden metastatic hormone sensitive prostate cancer: Long-term survival results from the STAMPEDE trial. Annals of Oncology. 2019;**30**(12):1992-2003

[50] Kyriakopoulos CE, Chen Y-H, Carducci MA, Liu G, Jarrard DF, Hahn NM, et al. Chemohormonal therapy in metastatic hormone-sensitive prostate cancer: Long-term survival analysis of the randomized phase III E3805 CHAARTED trial. Journal of Clinical Oncology. 2018;**36**(11):1080-1087

[51] Chi KN, Chowdhury S, Bjartell A, Chung BH, Gomes AJPS, Given R, et al. Apalutamide in patients with metastatic castration-sensitive prostate cancer: Final survival analysis of the randomized, double-blind, phase III TITAN study. Journal of Clinical Oncology. 2021;**39**(20):2294-2303

[52] Smith MR, Hussain M, Saad F, Fizazi K, Sternberg CN, Crawford ED, et al. Darolutamide and survival in metastatic. Hormone-Sensitive Prostate Cancer. 2022;**386**(12):1132-1142

[53] Fizazi K, Carles Galceran J, Foulon S, Roubaud G, McDermott R, Fléchon A, et al. LBA5 A phase III trial with a 2x2 factorial design in men with de novo metastatic castration-sensitive prostate cancer: Overall survival with abiraterone acetate plus prednisone in PEACE-1. Annals of Oncology. 2021;**32**:S1299

[54] Hadfield MJ, Lyall V, Holle LM, Dennison M. Updates in the treatment of non-metastatic castrate-resistant prostate cancer: The benefit of second-generation androgen receptor antagonists. Annals of Pharmacotherapy. 2023;**57**(11):1302-1311

[55] Petrylak DP, Tangen CM, Hussain MHA, Lara PN, Jones JA, Taplin ME, et al. Docetaxel and estramustine compared with mitoxantrone and prednisone for advanced refractory prostate cancer. The New England Journal of Medicine. 2004;**351**(15):1513-1520

[56] Ryan CJ, Smith MR, Bono JS, Molina A, Logothetis CJ, Souza P, et al. Abiraterone in metastatic prostate cancer without previous chemotherapy. The New England Journal of Medicine. 2013;**368**(2):138-148

[57] Beer TM, Armstrong AJ, Rathkopf DE, Loriot Y, Sternberg CN, Higano CS, et al. Enzalutamide in metastatic prostate cancer before chemotherapy. The New England Journal of Medicine. 2014;**371**(5):424-433

[58] Fizazi K, Scher HI, Molina A, Logothetis CJ, Chi KN, Jones RJ, et al. Abiraterone acetate for treatment of metastatic castration-resistant prostate cancer: Final overall survival analysis of the COU-AA-301 randomised, double-blind, placebo-controlled phase 3 study. The Lancet Oncology. 2012;**13**(10):983-992

[59] Scher HI, Fizazi K, Saad F, Taplin ME, Sternberg CN, Miller K, et al. Increased survival with enzalutamide in prostate cancer after chemotherapy. The New England Journal of Medicine. 2012;**367**(13):1187-1197

[60] de Wit R, de Bono J, Sternberg CN, Fizazi K, Tombal B, Wülfing C, et al. Cabazitaxel versus abiraterone or enzalutamide in metastatic prostate cancer. The New England Journal of Medicine. 2019;**381**(26):2506-2518

[61] Parker C, Nilsson S, Heinrich D, Helle SI, O'Sullivan JM, Fosså SD, et al. Alpha emitter radium-223 and survival in metastatic prostate cancer. The New England Journal of Medicine. 2013;**369**(3):213-223

[62] de Bono J, Mateo J, Fizazi K, Saad F, Shore N, Sandhu S, et al. Olaparib for metastatic castration-resistant prostate cancer. The New England Journal of Medicine. 2020;**382**(22):2091-2102

[63] Messina C, Giunta EF, Signori A, Rebuzzi SE, Banna GL, Maniam A, et al. Combining PARP inhibitors and androgen receptor signalling inhibitors in metastatic prostate cancer: A quantitative synthesis and meta-analysis. European Urology Oncology. 2024;**7**(2):179-188

Chapter 2

Histopathological Evaluation of Prostate Lesions: A Comprehensive Approach

Meeta Singh, Shabnam Singh, Nita Khurana, Neha Pandey, Vipul Ranjan Bhatt, Sophia Thomas, Tapan Jyoti Saikia, Shaad Sarvar Vali and Jennifer Kimnuntluangi

Abstract

This chapter encompasses the spectrum of prostatic diseases seen routinely in the evaluation of prostate biopsy or resection specimens. It covers the basic anatomy and histology, along with tissue examination and processing. The common benign conditions such as benign prostatic hyperplasia (BPH), various kinds of prostatitis, etc., are addressed briefly and prostate adenocarcinoma is discussed in a structured pattern, including the morphological variants, IHC, molecular profiling, microscopic variants, grading, mimickers, etc. Other rare tumors of the prostate are also discussed in brief. This chapter provides a comprehensive update on the 2022 WHO classification of urinary and male genital tumors.

Keywords: prostate, morphology, IHC, BPH, adenocarcinoma, mimics

1. Introduction

The prostate is a retroperitoneal organ that surrounds the bladder neck and prostatic urethra. In adults, it is funnel-shaped, weighs about 20 grams [1], and has its base beneath the bladder neck and apex above the urogenital diaphragm. Posteriorly, it is separated from the rectum by Denon Villiers fascia. It is divided into the anterior fibromuscular stroma and three distinct glandular zones, as proposed by Mc Neal (**Figure 1**) [2].

- The transition zone—envelopes the proximal prostatic urethra and comprises 5% of glandular tissue.
- The central zone—lies toward the base and contains the ejaculatory duct, which opens into the prostatic urethra at the verumontanum; comprises 20% of glandular tissue.
- The peripheral zone—envelopes the central and peripheral zones, and comprises most of the apex; it comprises approximately 70% of glandular tissue.

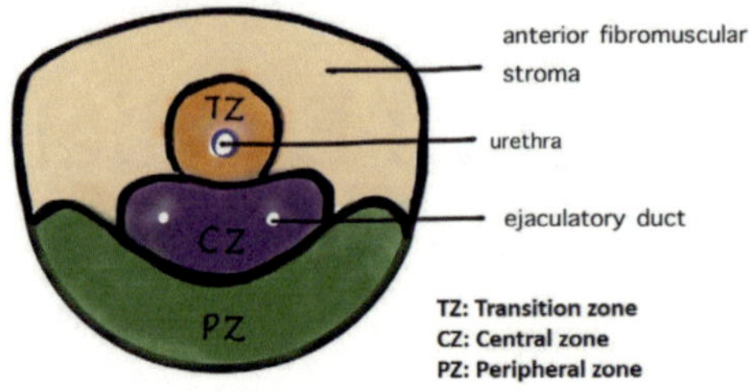

Figure 1.
Zones of the prostate gland.

These zones are at risk for different types of lesions; benign prostatic hyperplasia (BPH) primarily affects the transition zone, whereas carcinomas involve the peripheral zone. The prostate gland is partially surrounded by a fibrous capsule. The neurovascular bundles run posterolateral to the capsule bilaterally at 5 and 7 o'clock positions. Histologically, the prostate is comprised of glands separated by fibromuscular stroma. The glandular system consists of ducts and acini with little or no morphological difference. The glands often have papillary infoldings and undulating contour. The glands are lined by three types of cells:

- *Secretory cells*: They are located along the glandular lumen, columnar cells with relatively pale cytoplasm. They stain positively with prostate-specific antigen (PSA); prostate-specific acid phosphatase (PSAP); NKX3.1, some keratins but are negative for high molecular weight types like 34beta E12 [2, 3].

- *Basal cells*: They represent the stem cells and are located between the secretory cells and basement membrane; they are low cuboidal or cigar-shaped and may have prominent nucleoli. They express high molecular weight keratins like 34beta E12 and CK5/6; p63, p40 [2, 3]. Their presence helps to distinguish between benign conditions and well-differentiated carcinomas.

- *Neuroendocrine cells*: These cells are sparse and irregularly distributed with no proper known function.

The fibromuscular stroma consists of collagenous fibrous tissue and smooth muscle fibers. Inspissated secretions of the prostate may accumulate in some glands, forming spherical concretions known as corpora amylacea, which increase in number with age.

2. Tissue examination and processing

Prostate specimens received are mainly of three types: transrectal ultrasound (TRUS) biopsy; transurethral resection of prostate (TURP); resection specimens, that is, radical prostatectomy for tumors or suprapubic prostatectomy for benign hyperplasia.

2.1 TRUS needle biopsy

The number of cores is counted and measured (mm). Each core is submitted separately if labeled accordingly and processed. A minimum of three levels is to be examined.

2.2 TURP

Weigh and measure the dimensions of the prostatic chips received. Describe the chips, including color, consistency, and any abnormal area (hemorrhage or necrosis) if seen. As per College of American Pathologists (CAP) guidelines, specimens weighing 12 grams or less are entirely processed. For specimens weighing more than 12 grams, an additional 2 grams are required for every 5 grams of tissue beyond the initial 12 grams for processing [4, 5]. If carcinoma is detected and involves <5% of tissue, the remaining tissue should be entirely processed. In a previously diagnosed case of carcinoma, only a small amount of tissue can be processed.

2.3 Suprapubic prostatectomy

Weigh and measure (three dimensions, mm) the specimen. Serially section at 3–4 mm, carefully examine and describe, including color, consistency, any abnormal area, and areas of hemorrhage or necrosis. Submit at least eight sections from different areas.

2.4 Radical prostatectomy

Weigh the specimen and note the dimensions of the prostate and length of the attached seminal vesicle. Orient the specimen placing a probe through the urethra will help and paint the anterior, posterior, right lateral, left lateral, and superior and inferior surfaces using different colored inks. Cut the seminal vesicles and submit a section including the base of the vesicle with the prostate on both sides. The bladder neck margin (proximal) and apex (distal) are submitted. The remaining prostate is to be serially sectioned at 3–4 mm intervals and carefully examined. Note the color, consistency, any tumor nodule, area of hemorrhage, or necrosis. Sections are submitted from apex to base, and each slice can be bisected or quadrisected to fit the cassettes. All lymph nodes should be submitted after noting their number, size, and cut section appearance.

3. Benign prostatic hyperplasia

BPH is a nodular enlargement of prostate due to hyperplasia of both epithelial and stromal components. Incidence increases with increasing age, with >50% prevalence in males above 50 years of age, and is the most common benign prostatic disease in males above 50 years [1]. It is not a premalignant lesion. The precise etiology remains unclear, and no predisposing or protective factors have been identified other than castration [2, 3]. It is known to be an androgen-dependent disorder. Dihydrotestosterone (DHT), estrogens, and growth factors like fibroblast growth factor (FGF) and transforming growth factor (TGF) beta play an important role [2, 3]. The main symptoms include obstructive symptoms like hesitancy, weak urine stream, and post-micturition dribbling; irritative symptoms like frequency, urgency, and nocturia. Patient can also present with acute urinary retention requiring emergency catheterization for relief [1].

Grossly, the prostate gland is enlarged three to five times of normal or even more. On the cut section, it is seen to involve mainly the transition zone and thus encroach on the urethra, compressing it to a slit-like orifice. It has a multinodular appearance

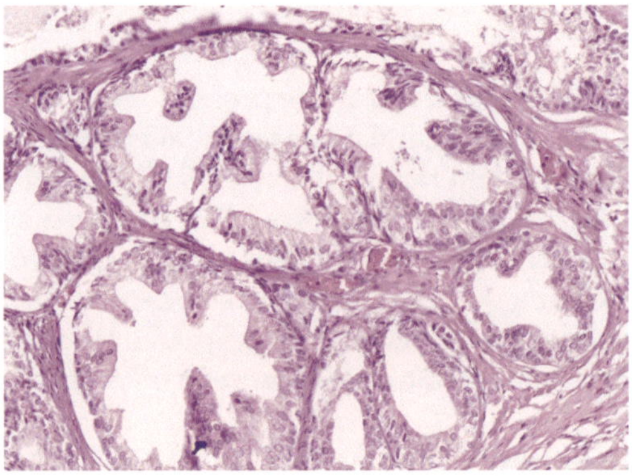

Figure 2.
BPH: Variable-sized ducts and acini lined by basal and secretory cells, H&E, 200x.

consisting of variable-sized nodules with a gray to yellow color. Microscopically, the earliest change is stromal proliferation, which is followed by glandular hyperplasia. The glandular component comprises variably sized acini and ducts lined by basal and secretory cells (**Figure 2**). The glands are dilated with papillary infoldings or cystic, and often contain corpora amylacea, which may be calcified. The epithelium is lined by flat to columnar cells. The stromal component comprises bland spindle cells with round to ovoid nuclei. Many morphologic variations exist, including clear cell cribiform hyperplasia, basal cell hyperplasia, adenosis, leiomyomatous nodules, fibroadenomatous, and phyllodes-type hyperplasia. Within areas of BPH, occasional lymphocytes are commonly seen, and a diagnosis of chronic prostatitis is not indicated due to its mere presence [2, 3].

4. Prostatitis

4.1 Bacterial prostatitis

Acute prostatitis is characterized by severe lower urinary tract symptoms (LUTS) including irritative and obstructive voiding symptoms with generalized urosepsis. Usually a self-limiting disease, acute prostatitis responds promptly to antibiotics. Chronic bacterial prostatitis is usually associated with mild to moderate pelvic pain and episodes of recurrent urinary tract infections (UTIs). As these infections are usually amenable to antimicrobial therapy, histologic examination of specimens removed for symptomatic prostatitis is thus uncommon. However, on histology, acute bacterial prostatitis is characterized by sheets of neutrophils within and around acini, intraductal desquamated cellular debris, and stromal edema and hyperemia.

4.2 Mycotic prostatitis

Fungal prostatic infections are relatively uncommon; however, the most common causes include blastomycesdermatitidis, Coccidioidesimmitis, and *Cryptococcus neoformans*. *Aspergillus fumigatus*, *Histoplasma capsulatum*, and *Candida albicans*, and *Candida glabrata* are among the other rarer causes (**Figure 3**) [2, 6]. Most fungal prostatitis occurs in the setting of urinary catheterization and use of broad-spectrum

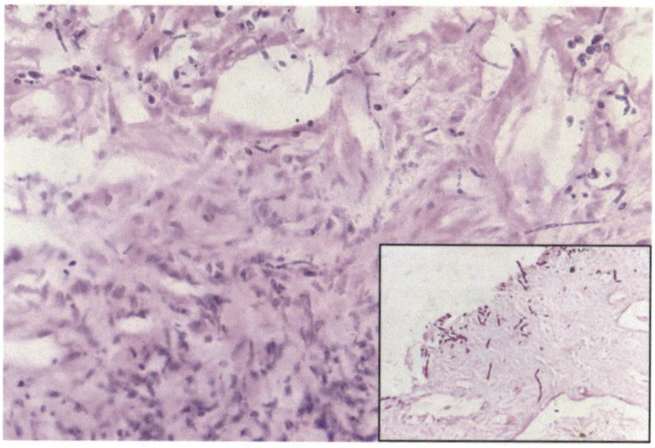

Figure 3.
Hyphae and budding yeast forms of candida, H&E stain, 400x, Inset: PAS stain, 400x.

antibiotics, leading to systemic hematogenous dissemination in immunocompromised and elderly hosts with comorbidities [2, 6].

4.3 Tuberculous prostatitis

Systemic tuberculous prostatitis is rare (incidence: 3–12%) due to timely diagnosis and treatment of disease for non-prostatic signs and symptoms of infection, as more than 90% of cases also show lung involvement [2]. However, infection might spread via hematogenous route or may directly invade from the urethra. Confluent areas of caseation, along with cavitation, may result in a grossly enlarged prostate with multiple cavities. Infection might spread to the urinary bladder and further to the rectum, perineum, and peritoneal cavity. The serum PSA levels may be increased. Bacillus Calmette-Guérin (BCG) immunotherapy for superficial urothelial cancer of the bladder may also result in the development of granulomas, which may vary from small, noncaseating and superficial to large, caseating, and throughout the prostate.

4.4 Nonspecific granulomatous prostatitis

Nonspecific granulomatous prostatitis is a rare disorder resulting from a localized immune-mediated reaction to ruptured prostatic secretions and contents. Mostly occurs in glands with preexisting nodular hyperplasia. High-grade fever, urinary obstruction, and hard prostate on palpation constitute the clinical symptoms. The cut surface shows yellow granular nodularity. Microscopically, these nodules show aggregates of dense inflammatory infiltrate chiefly composed of lymphocytes, plasma cells, epithelioid cells, and histiocytes, which often obscure and efface ductal and acinar elements (**Figure 4**). The early lesions show a tubercle-like reaction with multinucleated giant cells, neutrophils, eosinophils, and detritus within the dilated ducts and acini, which may as well rupture focally, resulting in localized granulomatous and chronic inflammatory reactions; however, microorganisms and caseous necrosis are absent. In contrast, the granulomas in early infectious noncaseating prostatitis surround intact acini. There is dense fibrosis in older lesions, leading to a firm to stony-hard prostate on palpation, simulating carcinoma in about 30% of cases [3]. Serum PSA levels may also be elevated. Immunohistochemical (IHC) stains for histiocytes and T cells surrounding the damaged ducts may help to differentiate from carcinoma.

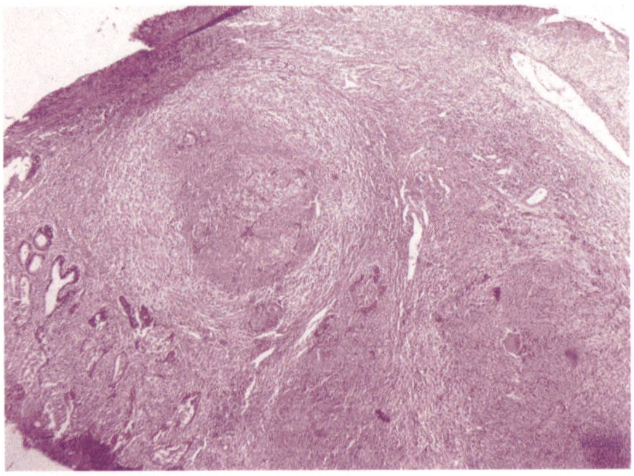

Figure 4.
Granulomatous prostatitis: nodules composed of dense inflammatory infiltrate chiefly comprising of lymphocytes, plasma cells, epithelioid cells, and histiocytes, with effacement of ductal and acinar elements, H&E, 40x.

4.5 Malakoplakia

Malakoplakia can rarely involve prostate, usually associated with primary bladder disease. It is believed to be caused by an impaired host response to bacterial infection, most commonly to *Escherichia coli* [2]. It is frequently seen in patients with either a primary or acquired immunodeficiency, such as diabetes, malignancy, or HIV/AIDS; a history of UTI strongly supports the diagnosis. In the prostate, malakoplakia can mimic carcinoma both clinically and radiologically. In needle core biopsy, there is periductal dense inflammatory infiltrate consisting mainly of histiocytes and scattered, atrophic prostatic glands along with basophilic cytoplasmic inclusions that have a targetoid appearance also known as Michaelis-Gutmann bodies.

5. Prostatic infarct

Prostatic infarcts remain mostly asymptomatic or sometimes may cause acute urinary retention due to edema. Serum PSAP and PSA may be elevated. Moore reported the incidence of infarcts to be 18–25% in carefully examined prostates [3]. They are usually associated with nodular hyperplasia, and the size and number of infarcts are directly proportional to the degree of hyperplasia. Other causes include trauma or infection due to cystitis, prostatitis, or a urinary catheter resulting in thrombosis of prostatic vessels. Grossly, they appear gray yellow, speckled, and size may vary from a few millimeters up to 5 cm. Microscopic sections show sharp areas of coagulative necrosis affecting glands and stroma; the latter may be spared sometimes in cases of nodular hyperplasia.

6. Calculi

The prostatic calculi are observed in about 7% cases of nodular hyperplasia and are composed of inorganic salts, namely phosphate salts of calcium, magnesium along with calcium carbonate and calcium oxalate [3]. The corpora amylacea, blood clots, bacteria, and dead epithelial cells act as nuclei for stone formation. They may get extremely hard, leading to suspicion of carcinoma on palpation. Their radiopaque nature makes them easily detectable on X rays.

7. Tumors of prostate

Table 1 describes the latest World Health Organization (WHO) classification of prostate tumors 2022.

7.1 High-grade prostatic intraepithelial neoplasia

Prostatic intraepithelial neoplasia (PIN) is considered to be the end of the spectrum of preinvasive proliferation of prostatic ducts and acini. The term PIN is now used interchangeably with high-grade PIN (HGPIN) as low-grade PIN are not routinely reported due to high inter-observer variability, poor reproducibility, and lack of definite association with prostatic carcinoma [8–12].

The only proven method to diagnose HGPIN is biopsy, as these lesions do not significantly raise the serum PSA level nor are easily detected on ultrasonography. The incidence of isolated HGPIN in the prostatic biopsy is about 9% in United States, with prevalence and volume of HGPIN rising proportionately with advancing age [10, 13, 14]. Hirori et al. [15] stated that African-American men have higher prevalence than whites in 50–60 age bracket, while Japanese have a lower incidence than men in the United States. This is in contrast to the study by Kilnk et al. [16] which showed that incidence of HGPIN is comparable in Asian and western men [16, 17].

Apart from HGPIN, which affects the peripheral zone, other precursors for prostate cancer include adenosis (atypical adenomatous hyperplasia), affecting the

1.	*Epithelial tumors of the prostate*	
	A.	**Glandular neoplasms of the prostate**
		• Prostatic cystadenoma • High-grade prostatic intraepithelial neoplasia • Intraductal carcinoma of the prostate • Prostatic acinar adenocarcinoma • Prostatic ductal adenocarcinoma • Treatment-related neuroendocrine prostatic carcinoma
	B.	Squamous neoplasms of the prostate
		• Adenosquamous carcinoma of the prostate • Squamous cell carcinoma of the prostate • Adenoid cystic (basal cell) carcinoma of the prostate
2.	*Mesenchymal tumors unique to the prostate*	
	Stromal tumors of the prostate	
		• Prostatic stromal tumor of uncertain malignant potential • Prostatic stromal sarcoma

Table 1.
WHO classification of prostate tumors [7].

transition zone and less likely for malignant transformation, and proliferative inflammatory atypia (PIA) [16, 18], which occurs frequently in the peripheral zone and has been shown to be in continuum with HGPIN and progress to a small adenocarcinoma lesion [19].

PIN mimics malignancy, cytologically exhibiting nuclear and nucleolar enlargement and cellular proliferations within preexisting ducts and acini. There is increased microvascular density in the stroma, which is intermediate between benign and malignant, along with loss of polarity (**Figure 5**) [8]. Tufting (most common), micropapillary, cribriform, and flat are the four primary histologic patterns of HGPIN that have been reported [18, 20]. Rarer patterns include signet ring cell, small cell neuroendocrine, mucinous, micro-vacuolated, and hobnail (inverted) pattern. The architectural patterns do not appear to differ in any way that is clinically significant, and identifying them seems to be only useful for diagnostic purposes.

The first signs of carcinoma, known as early stromal invasion, appear at the locations of basal cell breakdown and acinar outpouching in acini with HGPIN. About 2% of PIN's high-power tiny fields have this kind of microinvasion, which occurs equally frequently in all architectural forms. In concordance with cancer, HGPIN is typically multicentric and primarily located in the peripheral zone of the prostate. With an increase in pathologic stage, Gleason grade, positive surgical margins, and perineural invasion (PNI) in prostate cancer, the amount of HGPIN also increases, highlighting the association between PIN and cancer [14].

Basal cell markers such as p63 and high molecular weight keratins (HMWK) have shown promising results to rule out HGPIN from its mimickers, such as basal cell hyperplasia, inflammatory acini, atypical adenomatous hyperplasia, post-atrophic hyperplasia, and alteration in radiation therapy [21, 22].

HGPIN has been associated with more than 50 genetic and molecular disorders. Both HGPIN and prostate cancer have been linked to at least 10 of these alterations. Up to 79% cases of prostate cancer exhibit TMPRSS2-ERG gene fusion [23]. Up to 19% of HGPIN display the same fusion too, which has helped establish that HGPIN is the precursor state of cancer [24, 25]. A regulatory protein for mTOR, 14–3-3σ is over expressed in both HGPIN and prostate cancer [26]. Micro-satellite instability (MSI) and a positive Replication error phenotype (RER+) was seen to be present more in prostate cancer than PIN lesions [27]. FAS (fatty acid synthetase) and p53 expression

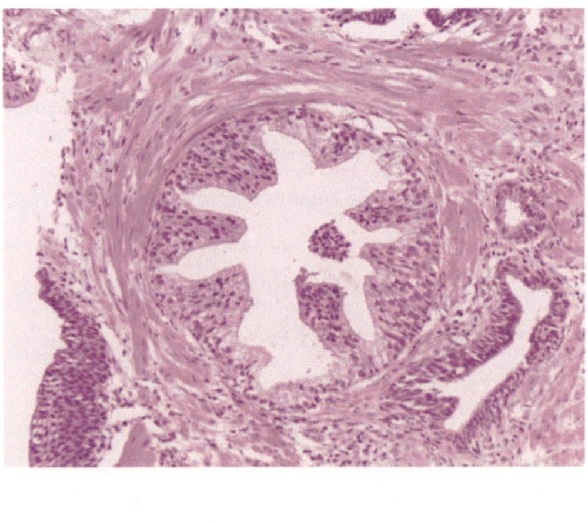

Figure 5.
Micropapillary pattern of HGPIN. Large duct with amphophilic cytoplasm, enlarged hyperchromatic nuclei and prominent nucleoli, H&E, 200x.

was also seen more in PIN and Prostate cancers than in normal tissues [28]. Bcl2 has been reported to be expressed in both low- and high-grade PIN [29].

Chromosomal anomalies such as gain of chromosome—8,10,7,12 and Y or loss of heterozygosity of chromosome 8p12–21, telomerase activation in some foci and epigenetic events such as hypermethylation has been seen in HGPIN [30–33]. Other markers include HER2/neu, c-erb-3 oncoproteins, c-met-proto-oncogene, inducible nitric oxide synthase, alpha-methylacyl-CoA racemase, glycoprotein A-80, apolipoprotein-D, and p16INK4A [34–37]. The finding of PIN in biopsy warrants further search for synchronous invasive carcinoma. A follow-up biopsy should be done at 3–6 months for 2 years and thereafter yearly for the rest of life.

7.2 Prostatic adenocarcinoma

The prostatic adenocarcinomas are usually present in males older than 65 years of age but may be seen in younger men as well. Clinical presentation includes dysuria, weak or interrupted flow of urine, nocturia, bladder or fecal incontinence, hematuria or hematospermia, painful ejaculation, erectile dysfunction, pain in the back, hips, or pelvis along with nonspecific symptoms of malignancy such as cancer cachexia [1, 38].

7.2.1 Prostatic acinar adenocarcinoma (conventional adenocarcinoma)

This cancer accounts for nearly all prostatic adenocarcinomas. The acini cells line the prostate's fluid-secreting glands. The cancer starts growing in the periphery of the prostate near the rectum, resulting in the late occurrence of urinary symptoms. It remains relatively indolent, and patients survive a long time after the diagnosis. Asymptomatic tumors are detected by digital rectal examination or by increased PSA levels. Local spread of adenocarcinoma occurs through extraprostatic extension or seminal vesicle invasion. Distant metastasis occurs when carcinoma invades the lymphovascular spaces. The most common sites of metastasis are regional pelvic lymph nodes, bones, and lungs. Rare sites include the liver and the testis [1, 39].

Grossly, the tumor is firm, gritty, and less spongy than surrounding non-neoplastic prostate [1]. Microscopically, there is haphazard proliferation of crowded, uniform small acini with irregular contours arranged in back-to-back fashion showcasing an infiltrative pattern. The acini are lined by a single layer of epithelial cells, and the basal cell layer is absent. The epithelial cells are cuboidal or columnar and have abundant amphophilic cytoplasm along with pleomorphic nuclei with the presence of one or more prominent macronucleoli. The presence of mitotic figures is according to the grade of the tumor. Corpora amylacea is rare. Intraluminal crystalloids, blue mucin, glomerulations, collagenous micronodules, and circumferential perineural invasion are some of the other features found in this carcinoma [1, 39, 40]. The unusual histological patterns include:

- *Atrophic adenocarcinoma (including aberrant p63 +)*: There is glandular proliferation with an infiltrative growth pattern; neoplastic cells have large nuclei with prominent nucleoli; glands lack basal cell layer. Many glands have scant cytoplasm, non-lobular, and infiltrative appearances on low power. High power shows some glands with abundant cytoplasm and other glands with scant cytoplasm (atrophic) but with an infiltrative architecture [39–41].

- *Pseudohyperplastic adenocarcinoma*: It occurs in the transition zone. Two of the following patterns are observed on low power:

a. Crowded glands lined by pseudostratified epithelium having rounded nuclei and a prominent nucleolus.

b. Large acini: Features associated with prostatic neoplasia, such as intraluminal crystalloids, pink amorphous secretions, and wispy blue mucin, are seen in a few cases. Discovery of intraluminal crystalloids at low magnification in hyperplastic-appearing glands may provide a diagnostic clue as to the presence of pseudohyperplastic carcinoma. It may be underdiagnosed because the pseudostratified epithelium looks like hyperplasia or HGPIN [39–41].

- *Microcystic adenocarcinoma*: It exhibits gland dilatation with intermediate-sized glands that are 10 times the size of usual small acinar adenocarcinoma glands. The expansion of the luminal spaces generates a rounded profile, and the luminal cell lining layer is flat, with or without atrophic changes. Intraluminal crystalloids and blue mucin are uniformly present. There is always admixture with usual small acinar adenocarcinoma, which most often comprises the majority of the tumor [39–41].

- *Foamy gland adenocarcinoma*: There is the presence of small glands with tall and columnar tumor cells, along with the occurrence of abundant foamy cytoplasm, luminal secretions, and bland nuclei. Occasionally, consist of cribriform, fused, or poorly formed glands, cords, single cells, or solid sheets. Gleason pattern 4 or 5. Can be underdiagnosed on a core biopsy [39–41].

- *Mucinous (colloid) adenocarcinoma*: Cut surface is mucinous/glistening. Uncommon variant. There is presence of extracellular mucin in at least 25% of tumors. Neoplastic cells having a variable degree of cytological atypia and glands float within lakes of extracellular mucin. The cribriform pattern is the most common, showing mucin within the gland lumina and dissecting between stromal muscle fibers. It is considered Gleason grade 4, showing aggressive biological behavior [39, 40].

7.2.1.1 Subtypes of prostatic acinar adenocarcinoma

a. *Signet ring-cell like adenocarcinom*: At least 25% of tumors consist of cells with a cytoplasmic vacuole that displaces the nucleus to the side (signet ring cell morphology). The cells, arranged mainly in small nests, diffusely infiltrate the stroma and invade the perineural and vascular spaces as well as the capsule of the prostate [42].

b. *Pleomorphic giant cell adenocarcinoma (PGCC)*: It is an aggressive form of prostatic adenocarcinoma. PGCC is defined by extreme nuclear atypia and pleomorphism, with characteristic bizarre multinucleated and mononuclear giant cells, usually with abundant cytoplasm and often atypical mitoses. Additional clinicopathologic features are perineural and/or lymphovascular invasion, cribriform architecture, and/or intraductal carcinoma or tumor necrosis [43].

c. *Sarcomatoid carcinoma*: Biphasic tumor with carcinomatous and spindle sarcomatoid components. The sarcomatoid areas are composed of spindle cells with large, pleomorphic, hyperchromatic nuclei and a high mitotic rate [39, 40].

d. *PIN-like carcinoma*: Rare tumors characterized by crowded, often cystically dilated glands architecturally resembling HGPIN, lined by malignant pseudostratified columnar epithelium. In some cases, the pseudostratified neoplastic epithelial cells are elongated, whereas in other cases the cells are cuboidal and nuclei are rounded with prominent nucleoli that are variably present. The histologic features overlap with pseudohyperplastic subtype [44]. According to WHO 2022, PIN-like carcinoma is classified as a subtype of acinar adenocarcinoma (although it can be related morphologically to ductal adenocarcinoma as well) [7].

7.2.2 Prostatic ductal adenocarcinoma

This cancer is a rarer but more aggressive form of adenocarcinoma. It develops in the cells lining the tubes and ducts of the prostate gland. It frequently develops along with acinar adenocarcinoma. It may not necessarily increase PSA levels, making it harder to detect. It may have papillary or polypoid mass extending into the urethra. *Prostatic ductal adenocarcinoma* (PDA) consists of large glands composed of tall columnar cells, which often have pseudostratified nuclei. The main patterns include cribriform, papillary, solid, and PIN-like pattern. The cribriform and papillary architecture are composed of pseudostratified columnar cells along with the occasional presence of comedo necrosis. The neoplastic cells have atypically large nuclei with coarse chromatin and large nucleoli. Mitotic figures are persistent. Considered Gleason grade 4 (or 5 if comedo necrosis present). The cribriform pattern in ductal adenocarcinoma has been shown to be more likely to have extraprostatic extension, seminal vesicle invasion, lymphovascular invasion, and advanced pathologic stage [39, 40].

7.2.3 Immunohistochemistry

Immunohistochemistry (IHC) offers limited utility in prostate adenocarcinomas as the diagnosis is based primarily on histomorphological features. Its application is known for enhancing the diagnostic accuracy mainly for prostate biopsies or identifying metastatic prostatic cancers in other organs [45]. During the interpretation of IHC markers, clinical, radiological, and histomorphological details should always be kept in mind. The use of these markers is mainly warranted in certain specific conditions, namely:

7.2.3.1 Diagnosis of minimal adenocarcinoma on needle biopsies

Small adenocarcinomas (measuring <1 mm or involving <5% of needle core tissue) form one of the most common adjunctive studies for use of IHC markers against basal cells [46, 47]. The most widely used immunomarkers for this purpose are high-molecular-weight cytokeratins (HMWCK) such as 34bE12 and p63. p40 which is an isoform of p63 is comparable for identifying basal cells. It is noteworthy that the loss of basal cells is not specific for carcinoma and may also be observed in benign pseudoneoplastic conditions like atrophy and adenosis [47, 48].

AMACR (also called P504S and racemase) is an α-methylacyl-CoA racemase that plays a role in the beta-oxidation of branched-chain fatty acids and fatty acid derivatives [49]. It shows positivity in prostatic adenocarcinoma with a high sensitivity and specificity. Of all cases, 80–100% of acinar adenocarcinomas show positivity, with characteristic granular cytoplasmic staining, sometimes with luminal accentuation. It also shows positive staining in most cases of HGPIN and thus cannot distinguish between invasive and noninvasive epithelium. This warrants the need for its use in conjunction with basal cell markers. In an ideal world, a malignant gland should show luminal reactivity for P504S in the luminal cells and absence of staining for the two basal cell markers, whereas the opposite should be true for benign glands. Another antibody named ERG protein expression shows high specificity for neoplastic prostatic glandular epithelium, but its sensitivity is only about 50% and does not add value beyond basal cell markers and AMACR expression for diagnosing minimal adenocarcinoma [50].

7.2.3.2 Distinction between poorly differentiated prostatic carcinoma and urothelial carcinoma

The best immunomarkers to aid in this differential diagnosis are PSA and GATA3 [46]. PSA is positive in 90–95% of high-grade adenocarcinomas of the prostate and negative in urothelial carcinomas whereas GATA3, a zinc finger transcription factor shows positivity in 80% of high-grade urothelial carcinomas and is almost always negative in prostatic adenocarcinoma. Other markers to confirm prostate origin are NKX3.1 (a homeobox-containing transcription factor), p501S, PSAP, and PSMA [46].

7.2.3.3 Differentiation of high-grade adenocarcinoma of the prostate from granulomatous prostatitis/xanthoma

The differential of a xanthoma or granulomatous prostatitis may arise in certain histological variants, such as the foamy gland variant of adenocarcinoma. The use of epithelial markers such as AE1/AE3 and CAM5.2, which show positivity for prostatic adenocarcinoma cells along CD68-staining histiocytes, will help in this distinction.

7.2.3.4 Differentiating between high-grade adenocarcinoma of the prostate and urinary bladder adenocarcinoma

The markers for high-grade prostatic adenocarcinoma are PSA, PSAP, and prostein. PSA and PSAP antibodies show high sensitivities (90–95%) for high-grade prostatic adenocarcinomas (Gleason score 8–10). They generally do not react with bladder adenocarcinoma, but sometimes even these markers may show positive staining. Therefore, the use of CDX2 and carcinoembryonic agent (CEA) which show a sensitivity of 47–65% for bladder adenocarcinomas, along with prostate-specific markers, is recommended [46].

7.2.3.5 Discrimination of high-grade adenocarcinoma of the prostate from colorectal adenocarcinoma

Both prostatic adenocarcinomas and colorectal carcinomas show proclivity for older males, and thus colon carcinoma serves as an important differential diagnosis. CDX2 and villin show positivity for cells of colon carcinoma and should be applied in adjunct to PSA, PSAP, and PSMA [46].

7.2.3.6 Diagnosis of metastatic adenocarcinoma of the prostate

Immunomarkers that help in proving prostatic origin are PSA, PSAP, prostein, and NKX3.1 with each of the markers reproducing a sensitivity of >94% [46, 51]. The use of PSA and PSAP is limited, as their expression may be decreased after androgen deprivation therapy [52]. Also, PSA shows immunoreactivity in some salivary gland neoplasms, while PSAP shows positivity in both salivary gland neoplasms and neuroendocrine carcinomas. It is also interesting to note that some cases of urinary bladder adenocarcinomas have shown positivity for prostein, but the characteristic granular perinuclear staining is not seen [53]. These evidences prove that NKX3.1 is highly specific and thus most reliable for prostatic adenocarcinomas [51]. Prostate-specific markers of limited diagnostic utility are PSMA, ERG, AR, and AMACR due to low sensitivity and specificity.

7.2.4 Molecular profiling

Large-scale genomic studies done in the recent past, including The Cancer Genome Atlas (TCGA) have lended further insights in understanding the molecular landscape of somatic DNA alterations in prostate cancer [54–57]. The most common molecular alterations associated with the initiation of prostate cancers are *MYC* overexpression, shortening of telomeres, inactivation of *GSTP1* and other genes by CpG island hypermethylation, and gene fusions involving ETS transcription factors (*TMPRSS2::ERG).* Some genes, such as the PI3K, MYC, and p53 pathways are altered in sporadic prostate cancer, whereas the RAS-MAPK pathway has shown little evidence. Noteworthy oncogenic drivers in 25–50% cases are androgen-driven ETS factors, withTMPRSS2-ERG fusion being most common. Other members of the ETS family that serve as 3′ partners include ETV1, ETV4, ETV5, and FLI1 [58, 59]. The prevalence of these ETS rearrangements ranges from 27–79% [59].

Other cases of acinar adenocarcinoma of the prostate are driven by somatic mutations involving *FLU*, *SPOP*, *FOXA1*, or *IDH1* which are mutually exclusive with ETS rearrangements and with each other. Progression of the disease is mitigated by gain of 8q24 (including *MYC),* loss of *PTEN,* inactivation of *TP53*, and additional mutations and hypermethylation events. The association of these genetic alterations is associated with a worse prognosis and goes on to prove that genomic instability is central to the disease progression of prostate cancers [60, 61].

Metastatic prostate cancers initial sensitivity to androgen deprivation or androgen receptors (AR) blockade, yet most cases progress to castration-resistant prostate cancer. This transition is seen to have association with *AR* gene amplification, mutation, or rearrangement, and/or with the activation of AR splice variants [62, 63]. This concludes that AR remains a key driver of late-stage disease. About 20% of metastatic prostatic carcinomas harbor germline or somatic alterations in DNA repair genes involved in homologous recombination repair (HRR), mismatch repair, and other genes, such as *BRCA1*, *BRCA2*, *ATM*, *CHEK2*, *FANCI*, and *PALB2* [57, 64, 65]. These findings have prompted the current guideline recommendations for germline and/or somatic testing for DNA repair defects in men with aggressive primary tumors and in men presenting with metastatic prostate cancer [66, 67].

7.2.5 Grading

The Gleason system is widely accepted and preferred grading system throughout the world for prostate adenocarcinoma [68]. It has undergone several modifications over the past 50 years, most recently after the International Society of Urological Pathology (ISUP) consensus conferences in 2005, 2014, and 2019 and the 2019 white paper by the Genitourinary Pathology Society (GUPS) [69–72]. The major modification happened in its manner of grading going from traditional Gleason grading to the now accepted grade group (GG) system [70].

The system is based primarily on the pattern of growth of neoplastic glands on low-power magnification, where 5 patterns are described, with 1 showing maximum differentiation and 5 showing least differentiation (**Table 2**). Owing to the heterogeneous tumor differentiation, prostate cancers often exhibit more than one pattern. In the traditional grading system, the most common patterns (primary and secondary) were recorded to derive the Gleason score (GS), however, it has now been revised to the primary and worst patterns for biopsy. The sum of these patterns constitutes the Gleason score that ranges from 2 to 10 [73–75]. This grading does not consider nuclear and cytoplasmic features.

The 2005 ISUP consensus conference introduced a key number of changes, most noteworthy was Patterns 1 and 2 are no longer assigned to core needle biopsy specimens and are rarely used in radical prostatectomy (RP) specimens, leaving an effective range of 6–10 for Gleason scores.

Gleason pattern	Representative Diagram	Key morphological features	Comments
1 and 2	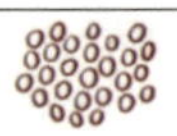	Discrete regular glands; circumscribed, rounded nodules	Not used for needle biopsy specimens; very rarely used in grading radical prostatectomy specimens
3	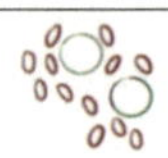	Discrete glands with marked variation in size and shape; infiltration between non-neoplastic acini Includes pseudohyperplastic, atrophic, and microcystic patterns	No longer includes cribriform or glomeruloid glands after the ISUP 2005 and 2014 consensus conferences
4	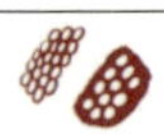	Fused microacinar glands, poorly formed glands without well-defined lumina, cribriform glands, or glomeruloid glands	
5	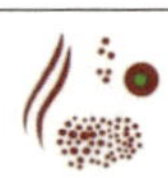	Minimal glandular differentiation, comprising solid sheets, cords, small solid cylinders, or single cells OR Solid, cribriform or papillary structures with central necrosis (comedocarcinoma)	

Table 2.
Gleason grade patterns (after the ISUP 2005 and 2014 modifications).

Also, since 2005 it is recommended to derive the GS by adding the primary pattern with the worst pattern for core needle biopsy, unlike radical prostatectomy specimens where the score is derived from the sum of the primary and secondary prevalent patterns [69]. Some radical prostatectomy specimens may show more than 2 patterns, where the worst pattern (pattern 5) represents the smallest volume, being referred to as the tertiary high-grade pattern. In such situations, if the tertiary grade pattern constitutes >5% of the tumor volume, it becomes the secondary pattern in Gleason scoring [71, 72, 76, 77]. Higher tertiary pattern volumes are associated with a worse prognosis and reported despite the 5% cut-off being somewhat arbitrary. If the higher-grade component constitutes <5% of the tumor, it is to be dealt differently in the 2019 ISUP and GUPS systems (**Table 3**).

In 2014 ISUP conference, the concept of grade groups (GG1-GG5) was endorsed. It is also referred to as "ISUP grade" or simply "WHO Classification of Tumors grade (WHO grade)" in order to separate it from the other grade grouping systems used before 2013. The most distinctive advantage is with respect to the communication of results to patients, clinicians, and researchers. This advantage can be understood by noting that Gleason score 3 + 3 = 6 cancers are assigned Gleason Grade Group (GG1) which highlights their generally favorable prognosis, whereas 3 + 4 = 7 cancers (GG2) are placed in a separate grade group compared to 4 + 3 = 7 cancers (GG3) highlighting the higher risk of recurrence associated with the latter (**Figures 6–8**; **Table 4**) [70, 78].

7.2.6 Serum prostate-specific antigen levels

PSA is secreted into the seminal fluid, where it is responsible for semen liquefaction. The release of PSA into the bloodstream enables the detection in serum. Serum PSA levels correlate with the risk of prostate cancer in most instances. When combined with patient age, digital rectal examination findings, and additional factors such as race and family history, serum PSA can be used to assess the need for biopsy.

The established normal range is 2–4 ng/ml [79]. The use of PSA for screening is limited as its levels can be raised in BPH and prostatitis, as well as with mechanical manipulation of the prostate gland. These factors, when coupled with the biological variation of PSA concentrations, result in its low specificity and low positive predictive value.

For improving the specificity of PSA testing, several PSA derivatives are now being used. These include *PSA density* (the ratio of PSA to gland volume), *PSA*

Issues		GUPS 2019 Recommendations	ISUP 2019 Recommendations
Minor/tertiary pattern in RP specimen	GP3 (25%), GP4, and GP5 pattern in RP present with GP5 < 5%	GS 3 + 4 = 7 or 4 + 3 = 7 with minor/tertiary pattern 5	
	> 95% GP3 with <5% GP4*	GS 3 + 4 = 7	GS 3 + 3 = 6 with minor/ tertiary pattern 4
	> 95% GP3 with <5% GP5*	GS 3 + 5 = 8	GS 3 + 3 = 6 with minor/ tertiary pattern 5
	> 95% GP4 with <5% GP5*	GS 4 + 5 = 9	GS 4 + 4 = 8 with minor/ tertiary pattern 5

Table 3.
Unresolved disagreements between GUPS and ISUP recommendations.

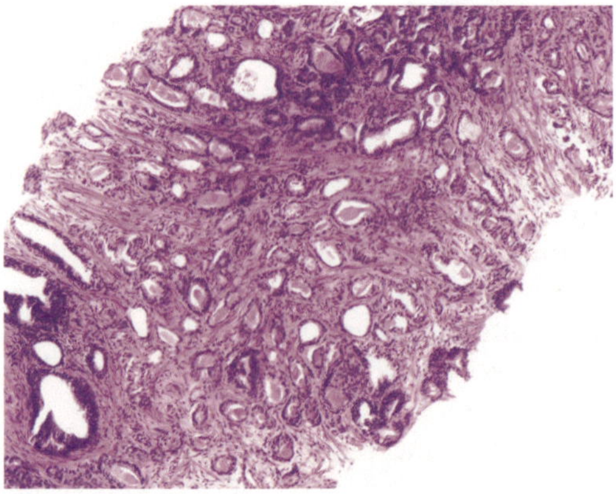

Figure 6.
Gleason grade 3 pattern showing well-formed glands with infiltration, H&E, 100x.

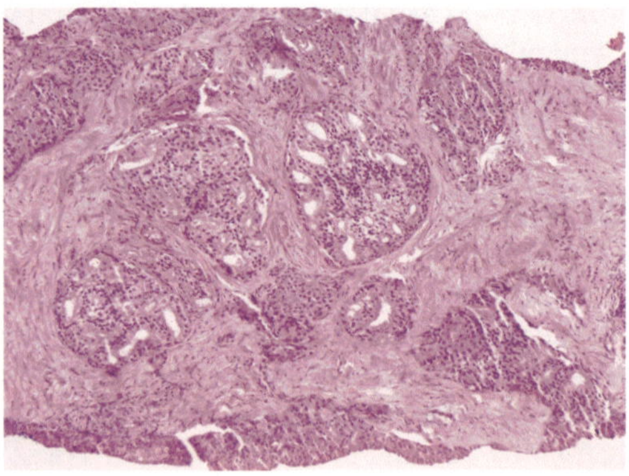

Figure 7.
Gleason grade 4 pattern showing ill-defined glands in a cribriform pattern, H&E, 100x.

doubling time, *PSA velocity* (the change of PSA over time), and age- and race specific PSA reference ranges. This step has resulted in modest improvements in the specificities in some studies [80, 81]. While these studies are potentially important, the results will remain underutilized unless they are able to provide information on how to address clinically relevant questions.

7.2.7 Metastasis

Hematogenous route is the most common mode of spread. Higher grade, larger primary and increase in local stage has been associated with increased likelihood of metastasis [82].

Bone (90%): Prostate cancers show predisposition for spread to bone, mainly due to the unique microenvironment and high vascularity (seed and soil hypothesis), although it is not universal [83]. Ten percent of new cases are identified after bony metastasis, while 70–80% of all the relapsed cases post radical prostatectomy also show bony metastasis [82]. Lesions are more osteoblastic than osteolytic. Multifocal small lesions in the axial skeleton, particularly in close proximity to bone marrow, are the most common pattern. Patients present either with cord compression symptoms,

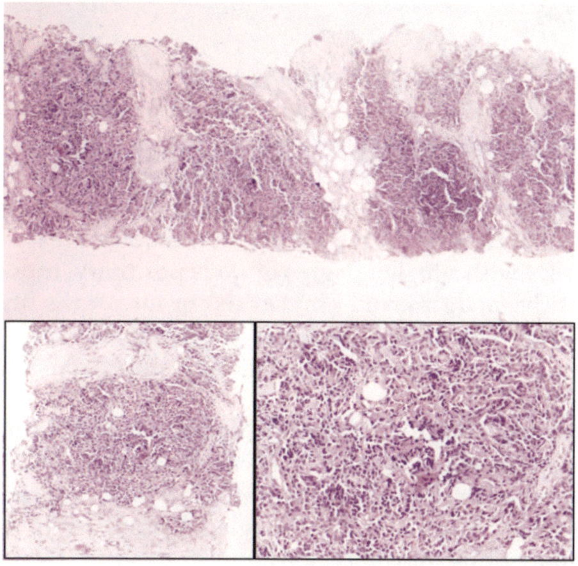

Figure 8.
Gleason grade 5 pattern showing single cell infiltration along with solid sheets, H&E, 40x, 100x (Inset- left) and 400x (Inset- right).

Grade Group	Gleason Score	Definition
1	6	Only individual, discrete, well-formed glands
2	3 + 4 = 7	Predominantly well-formed glands with lesser component of poorly formed/ fused/cribriform/glomeruloid glands
3	4 + 3 = 7	Predominantly poorly formed/fused/cribriform/glomeruloid glands with lesser component of well-formed glands
4	4 + 4 = 8, 3 + 5 = 8, 5 + 3 = 8	Only poorly formed/fused/cribriform/glomeruloid glands or Predominantly well-formed glands and lesser component lacking glands or Predominantly lacking glands with lesser component of well-formed glands
5	4 + 5 = 9, 5 + 4 = 9, 5+ 5 = 10	Lack of gland formation (or with necrosis) with or without poorly formed/fused/ cribriform glands

Table 4.
Histologic Definition of the Grade Groups.

or pathological fractures. The spine (lumbar vertebrae particularly), pelvis, and ribs are the most common sites of spread [82, 83].

Viscera: Lungs (45%), liver (25%), and pleura (21%) are the most common visceral organs involved, while others including peritoneum, adrenal, ureters, kidney, meninges, spleen, testis, etc., have been noted [83]. Neuroendocrine tumors have a propensity toward visceral metastasis compared to bone.

Node: Nodal metastasis is associated with high risk (10-year survival of 47–86%) and poor outcome. The location of the organ makes excision of the entire drainage network unfeasible. Most commonly, the regional pelvic nodes are involved, followed by paraaotic and mediastinal nodes [2].

7.2.8 Prognostic factors

Prostate cancer has one of the best survival rates, with a 5-year rate of 97% in the United States [84]. Survival time will be determined by multiple factors. Metastatic foci act as a sign of poor prognosis [82]. Others include:

Age: With advancing age (especially more than 65 years), tumors present at a higher stage and also have an increased risk of post-procedural complications [85].

Tumor volume: A study by McNeal et al. [85] correlated increased tumor burden (critical volume 12 cc) with a higher degree of node positivity, capsular breach, loss of differentiation, positive margins, and a higher risk of metastasis [85].

Zone of involvement: According to McNeal's Zones, cancers arising from the transitional zone have more favorable pathological features than those arising from the peripheral zone [85].

Heterogeneity and multicentricity: Multifocality is associated with a higher grade, stage, and recurrence compared to unifocal prostate cancer [85].

Grading: Gleason grade still is the strongest clinical predictor for cancer progression. A grade more than 7 is associated with higher risk of extra-prostatic extension, recurrence post-therapy, and mortality [85, 86].

PSA: Baseline and rapid rise of PSA levels have been well included in the risk estimations for the survivability of prostate cancer outcomes as well as for follow-up of patients post-therapy. High level of PSA has been a good screening tool to further evaluate patients for cancer. Rapid rise in post-therapy levels is a strong predictor for poor outcome [86].

Perineural invasion (PNI): PNI has been the major mechanism of extra-capsular extension by cancer cells in prostate. However, the amount of prognostic influence is debated upon (**Figure 9**) [86].

PIN: PIN has also been under conflicting reports regarding its influence in prognosis. A low-grade PIN is not reported. A high-grade PIN, in absence of carcinoma, may have an increased risk of detecting malignancy, however, in its presence, may not have any prognostic relevance [87].

Intraductal carcinoma: It is an independent prognostic risk factor for survival and is associated with high Gleason's Grade, larger tumor burden, and increased risk of metastasis [87].

Extra-prostatic extension: It has an independent poor prognostic outcome resulting in a higher progression rate and decreased survival [87].

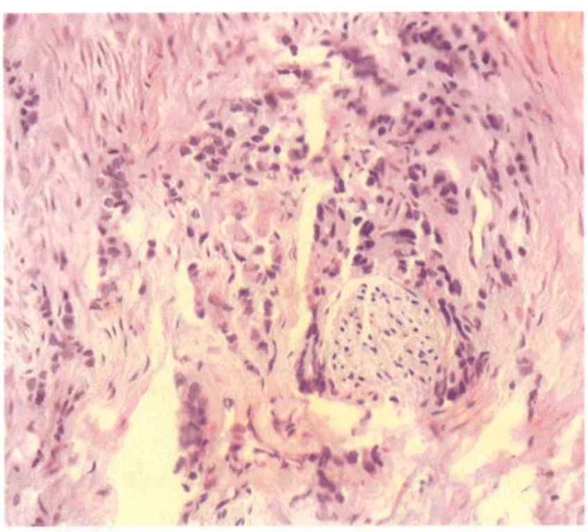

Figure 9.
PNI, H&E, 400x.

Positive margins: It is one of the most significant prognostic factors after grading of the tumor. A positive margin has been associated with biochemical recurrence of the cancer. Combined with Gleason's grade of the margin, the presence of any Grade 4/5 pattern has doubled the risk of biochemical recurrence than of Grade 3 [87].

Other biochemical prognostic factors: Low E cadherin expression, high IGF expression, p53 mutations, decreased p27 levels, high p21 levels, and high ploidy status are few of the biochemical parameters known to influence prognosis and decrease survivability of the patients. AR mutations have been a major cause of hormone therapy-resistant prostate cancer, decreasing survivability and increasing recurrence [85].

7.2.9 Mimickers of malignancy

1. *Prostatic atrophy:* Atrophic glands may have open lumina, crowded cells, scant cytoplasm, and an increased N:C ratio [2]. Post-atrophic hyperplasia will have an increased number of similar glands and less stroma. There can be isolated areas of increased proliferation, dilated glands surrounded by fibrosis, etc. Partial atrophy can show focal areas of crowding and disorganization with a mild increase in the N:C ratio. Gland-forming adenocarcinomas have basally situated nuclei and pale to amphophilic abundant cytoplasm, rather than scant. Basal markers are consistently negative; however, atrophy may show patchy negative in some areas. AMACR may be positive in those patchy basal-negative areas.

2. *Seminal vesicles/ejaculatory duct:* Edge of prostate cores may show the irregular glandular epithelium of seminal vesicle with luminal projection diverticulations and mild nuclear degenerative atypia. The presence of prominent lipofuchsin granules is an aid, although enlarged lysosomes in normal prostate glands may appear similar. Lipofuchsin-like granules are absent in cancer cells. Prostate markers are negative in seminal vesicles. The basal layer is intact in the seminal vesicle.

3. *Adenosis*: Adenosis, especially atypical adenomatous hyperplasia, can show numerous crowded pale staining glands, with focal conspicuous nucleoli resembling a nodule of low-grade adenocarcinoma. There is an abrupt transition from normal glands to malignant glands in carcinoma compared to the smoother transition in adenosis. Glands of adenocarcinoma are haphazardly arranged and infiltrate the stroma at right angles to each other, compared to the lobular arrangement of adenosis. Associated complexity of glands like branching, irregular shape, and papillary infolding are more features of benign disease than malignant. Basal cell markers are intact, at least focally, in adenosis.

4. *Sclerosing adenosis:* Small relatively localized foci of glands resembling ordinary adenosis, merging with cords and singly scattered cells with occasional conspicuous nucleoli. Hyalinized basement membrane-like component in a few glands. Prominent stromal component in sclerosing adenosis, absent in malignancy. Myoepithelial cell markers are absent in cancer.

5. *Others*:

Conditions simulating low grade (Gleason score 6): Cowper glands, radiation atypia, basal cell hyperplasia, nephrogenic adenoma, verumontanum hyperplasia, mesonephric hyperplasia.

Conditions simulating high grade (Gleason score 7–10): Nonspecific granulomatous prostatitis, paraganglia, clear cell cribriform hyperplasia, xanthoma, signet ring cell lymphocytes (degenerated or artifactual changes in lymphocytes).

7.3 Squamous cell carcinoma prostate

Squamous cell carcinoma prostate (SCC), accounts for less than 1% of all carcinomas of prostate [88]. The age at diagnosis ranges from 52 to 79 years [89]. The patients present with complaints of straining during micturition, weak stream, hesitancy, dysuria, infection, and bone pain due to metastases. Bony lesions in SCC, unlike prostatic adenocarcinoma, are osteolytic [90–92].

Numerous theories suggesting the neoplastic cell of origin of SCC include either basal or reserve cells of acini of prostate or transitional epithelium of urethra or ducts [93, 94]. Other theories explaining the histogenesis are: (1) adenocarcinoma cells undergoing metaplastic transformation; (2) a collision-type tumor, in which the squamous component develops from metaplastic foci following radiation or hormone therapy; and (3) a potential deviance from pluripotent stem cells with the capacity for multidirectional differentiation [95–98].

Mott et al. described the first approved criterion to determine the histologic characteristics of SCC, which consisted of the following: (1) an invasive disordered growth and cellular anaplasia that clearly indicated the presence of a malignant neoplasm; (2) distinct squamous features, such as keratinization, squamous pearls, and/or multiple distinct intercellular bridges; (3) no glandular or acinar pattern; (4) no history of estrogen therapy; and (5) the absence of SCC elsewhere, especially in the bladder [88]. In order to distinguish between SCC and non-neoplastic squamous metaplasia, which might result from radiation therapy, estrogen therapy, infarct, acute or chronic prostatitis, or granulomatous prostatitis caused by Bacillus-Calmette-Guérin, these parameters are crucial [99].

There is no specific and reliable IHC marker to differentiate between well-differentiated SCC from atypical squamous metaplasia or primary prostatic SCC from metastatic squamous cell carcinoma, as highlighted by Lager et al. [100] Clinically, the serum PSA and PAP levels remain unchanged [91]. SCC is an aggressive tumor with a mean survival of 14 months. Patients present with poorly differentiated grade in 45% cases and metastasis in 32% cases [101, 102].

7.4 Adenosquamous carcinoma

Adenosquamous carcinoma (ASCC) of prostate is a very rare form of prostatic carcinoma, with an incidence of 0.03 cases per million; it is even rarer than squamous cell carcinoma of prostate [103]. Patients present with dysuria, pain in rectum or pelvis, urinary retention, infection, hematuria, or bone pain as a result of metastases.

ASCC are composed of both glandular and squamous components with the squamous component accounting for an average of 40% tumor [5–95%] [104]. In a study conducted by Jue et al., it was seen that the majority of the patients with ASCC had poor or undifferentiated histology. The histogenesis of ASCC of the prostate can be understood by a number of theories: (i) adenocarcinoma cells undergoing metaplastic transformation; (ii) collision-type tumor; (iii) Pluripotent stem cells with the ability to differentiate in several directions represent the source of ASCC; (iv) Clonal evolution or divergence of persistent cancer, related to the selective pressure of therapy, would be a more likely explanation for ASCC occurring after radiation or androgen deprivation therapy [96, 105–109]. Glandular cells are positive for PSA, PAP, low molecular weight keratin (LMWK), and negative for high molecular weight keratin (HMWK), while the squamous component show positive staining HMWK and negative for LMWK, PAP, and PSA [96]. The molecular mechanism of this neoplasm is poorly understood. DNA analysis of ASCC has shown that the adenocarcinoma component was diploid and the squamous component was aneuploid and tetraploid [107]. The disease typically spreads by metastases, most commonly to lymph nodes and bones. The prognosis is dismal, with the expected median survival time to be only 12–14 months.

7.5 Adenoid cystic carcinoma prostate

Also known as basaloid carcinoma or adenoid cystic-like tumor, adenoid cystic carcinoma prostate (ACC) of prostate is a rare yet unique variant (incidence: 0.01%) that shares similar histomorphology to its salivary gland counterpart. They have insidious onset with recurrent and metastatic potential, as shown by few studies. The patients complain of obstructive symptoms or hematuria [110, 111]. The age bracket extends from 28 to 97 years and a peak between 60 and 75 years. Serum analysis yields a near normal serum PSA level. Patients in whom serum PSA level was raised were invariably found to have foci of prostatic adenocarcinoma. These findings suggest the difference in cell of origin of ACC, which are the non-secretory basal cells, and the importance of histomorphological and immunohistochemical staining in the diagnosis of these cases [112].

ACC can be divided histologically into basaloid type or adenoid cystic type. The basaloid variant shows irregular, variably sized solid nests, cords, and trabeculae exhibiting peripheral palisading of basaloid cells, with individual cells showing pleomorphism, a high N:C ratio, an irregular nucleus, and infiltration of adjacent structures. There is minimal or absent cribriform arrangement in these types of lesions [112]. The adenoid cystic variant is identified by prominent cribriform architecture, hyalinized, eosinophilic, or mucinous stroma with mucoid secretion in the lumen [113].

7.6 Mesenchymal tumors of prostate

Leiomyoma is the most common benign mesenchymal tumor of prostate. However, it lacks the well-organized fascicles and does not show degenerative features such as hyalinization, necrosis, or calcification [114].

Sarcomas of prostate are classified as prostatic stromal tumor of uncertain malignant potential (STUMP) and prostatic stromal sarcoma (PSS) based on degree of stromal cellularity, presence of mitotic figures, necrosis, and stromal overgrowth. They typically present with lower urinary tract obstruction and less commonly with a palpable mass, hematuria, hematospermia, or rectal fullness. They typically occur in the transition and peripheral zones of the prostate. The median age of presentation of STUMP is 57.5 years, which is slightly older than that of PSS, which is 51.5 years [115].

STUMP has five histological patterns: (1) hypercellular atypical stromal cells with a degenerative appearance, (2) hypercellular bland fusiform stromal cells, (3) phyllodes pattern, (4) myxoid stroma containing bland stromal cells, (5) epithelioid stromal pattern. It is positive for vimentin and PR, variably positive for CD34, SMA, and desmin, and uncommonly expresses ER. KIT, S100, and STAT6 are negative. It can be differentiated from Florid BPH by an extensive growth of atypical stromal cells and an absence of nodularity and thick-walled vessels [115].

PSS is rare, accounting for <1% of prostatic cancers. It may be circumscribed or may infiltrate surrounding benign prostate glands. It shows diffuse stromal growth in storiform, epithelioid, fibrosarcomatous, or leaf-like patterns or can be patternless also. It often presents with diffuse stromal hypercellularity, cytological atypia, increased or atypical mitosis, and necrosis. It is positive for vimentin and variably positive for CD34, while usually negative for SMA and desmin and uncommonly expresses ER and PR. Epithelial markers like pancytokeratin are rarely positive. It has the potential to act aggressively and can metastasize to distant sites such as bone and lung [115].

8. Conclusion

Prostatic parenchyma is known to show a variety of non-neoplastic and neoplastic pathologies. Being a retroperitoneal organ, a limited prostatic specimen is acquired via various guided methods or via complete organ excision. Much of the benign pathologies like BPH and prostatitis are well managed conservatively and have a good prognosis. Carcinomas of the prostate are the most common type of primary prostatic malignancy, with specific precursor lesions such as PIN. Recent advancements in molecular profiling have shed light on the genomic instability that drives prostatic adenocarcinoma. Key alterations, particularly in the androgen receptor gene, play a critical role in the transition to castration-resistant prostate cancer. The identification of TMPRSS2-ERG gene fusions and other molecular markers has significantly enhanced our understanding of tumor behavior, paving the way for personalized therapeutic strategies.

Author details

Meeta Singh*, Shabnam Singh, Nita Khurana, Neha Pandey, Vipul Ranjan Bhatt, Sophia Thomas, Tapan Jyoti Saikia, Shaad Sarvar Vali and Jennifer Kimnuntluangi
Maulana Azad Medical College and Associated Lok Nayak Hospital, New Delhi, India

*Address all correspondence to: meetamamc@gmail.com

IntechOpen

© 2024 The Author(s). Licensee IntechOpen. This chapter is distributed under the terms of the Creative Commons Attribution License (http://creativecommons.org/licenses/by/4.0), which permits unrestricted use, distribution, and reproduction in any medium, provided the original work is properly cited.

References

[1] Netto G, J, Amin MB. The lower urinary tract and male genital system. In: Kumar V, Abbas AK, Aster JC, editors. Robbins and Cotran Pathologic Basis of Disease. 10th ed. Philadelphia: Elsevier; 2018. pp. 953-983

[2] Epstein JI, Netto GJ. Prostate and seminal vesicles. In: Longacre TA, Greenson JK, Hornick JL, Reuter VE, editors. Mills and Sternberg's Diagnostic Surgical Pathology. 7th ed. Philadelphia, PA: Wolters Kluwer; 2022. pp. 2305-2350

[3] McKenney J, K. Prostate and seminal vesicles. In: Goldbum JR, Lamps LW, McKenney JK, Myers JL, editors. Rosai and Ackerman's Surgical Pathology. 11th ed. Philadelphia: Elsevier; 2018. pp. 1097-1134

[4] O'Rourke D, M, Allen DC. Prostate. In: Allen DC, Cameron RL, editors. Histopathology Specimens: Clinical, Pathological, and Laboratory Aspects. 2nd ed. London: Springer; 2013. pp. 307-318

[5] Loda B, MF, Welch WR. Genitourinary specimens. In: Lester SC, editor. Manual of Surgical Pathology. 3rd ed. Philadelphia: Elsevier; 2010. pp. 384-419

[6] Singh S, Singh M, Bains L, Sagar T. Candida prostatitis: A rare entity. Tropical Doctor. 2023;**53**(2):282-284

[7] WHO Classification of Tumours Editorial Board. WHO Classification of the Urinary and Male Genital Tumours. 5th ed. Lyon, France: WHO Classification of Tumours Editorial Board; 2022

[8] Bostwick DG, Qian J. High-grade prostatic intraepithelial neoplasia. Modern Pathology. 2004;**17**(3):360-379

[9] Morote J, Schwartzmann I, Celma A, Roche S, de Torres IM, Mast R, et al. The current recommendation for the management of isolated high-grade prostatic intraepithelial neoplasia. BJU International. 2022;**129**(5):627-633

[10] Argani P, Epstein JI. Inverted (hobnail) high-grade prostatic intraepithelial neoplasia (PIN): Report of 15 cases of a previously undescribed pattern of high-grade PIN. The American Journal of Surgical Pathology. 2001;**25**(12):1534-1539

[11] Epstein JI, Carmichael M, Partin AW. OA-519 (fatty acid synthase) as an independent predictor of pathologic stage in adenocarcinoma of the prostate. Urology. 1995;**45**(1):81-86

[12] McNeal JE, Bostwick DG. Intraductal dysplasia: A premalignant lesion of the prostate. Human Pathology. 1986;**17**(1):64-71

[13] Sakr WA, Sarkar FH, Sreepathi P, Drozdowicz S, Crissman JD. Measurement of cellular proliferation in human prostate by AgNOR, PCNA, and SPF. The Prostate. 1993;**22**(2):147-154

[14] Jenkins RB, Qian J, Lieber MM, Bostwick DG. Detection of c-myc oncogene amplification and chromosomal anomalies in metastatic prostatic carcinoma by fluorescence in situ hybridization. Cancer Research. 1997;**57**(3):524-531

[15] Hiroi H, Inoue S, Watanabe T, Goto W, Orimo A, Momoeda M, et al. Differential immunolocalization of estrogen receptor alpha and beta in rat ovary and uterus. Journal of Molecular Endocrinology. 1999;**22**(1):37-44

[16] Klink JC, Miocinovic R, Galluzzi CM, Klein EA. High-grade

prostatic intraepithelial neoplasia. Korean Journal of Urology. 2012;**53**(5):297

[17] Desai SB, Borges AM. The prevalence of high-grade prostatic intraepithelial neoplasia in surgical resection specimens: An Indian experience. Cancer: Interdisciplinary International Journal of the American Cancer Society. 2002;**94**(9):2350-2352

[18] De Marzo AM, Haffner MC, Lotan TL, Yegnasubramanian S, Nelson WG. Premalignancy in prostate cancer: Rethinking what we know. Cancer Prevention Research. 2016;**9**(8):648-656

[19] Wang W, Bergh A, Damber JE. Morphological transition of proliferative inflammatory atrophy to high-grade intraepithelial neoplasia and cancer in human prostate. The Prostate. 2009;**69**(13):1378-1386

[20] Cheville JC, Reznicek MJ, Bostwick DG. The focus of "atypical glands, suspicious for malignancy" in prostatic needle biopsy specimens: Incidence, histologic features, and clinical follow-up of cases diagnosed in a community practice. American Journal of Clinical Pathology. 1997;**108**(6):633-640

[21] Novis DA, Zarbo RJ, Valenstein PA. Diagnostic uncertainty expressed in prostate needle biopsies: A College of American Pathologists Q-probes study of 15 753 prostate needle biopsies in 332 institutions. Archives of Pathology and Laboratory Medicine. 1999;**123**(8):687-692

[22] Yang XJ, Lecksell K, Gaudin P, Epstein JI. Rare expression of high-molecular-weight cytokeratin in adenocarcinoma of the prostate gland: A study of 100 cases of metastatic and locally advanced prostate cancer. The American Journal of Surgical Pathology. 1999;**23**(2):147-152

[23] Tomlins SA, Rhodes DR, Perner S, Dhanasekaran SM, Mehra R, Sun XW, et al. Recurrent fusion of TMPRSS2 and ETS transcription factor genes in prostate cancer. Science. 2005;**310**(5748):644-648

[24] Perner S, Mosquera JM, Demichelis F, Hofer MD, Paris PL, Simko J, et al. TMPRSS2-ERG fusion prostate cancer: An early molecular event associated with invasion. The American Journal of Surgical Pathology. 2007;**31**(6):882-888

[25] Mosquera JM, Perner S, Genega EM, Sanda M, Hofer MD, Mertz KD, et al. Characterization of TMPRSS2-ERG fusion high-grade prostatic intraepithelial neoplasia and potential clinical implications. Clinical Cancer Research. 2008;**14**(11):3380-3385

[26] Evren S, Dermen A, Lockwood G, Fleshner N, Sweet J. mTOR–RAPTOR and 14-3-3σ immunohistochemical expression in high grade prostatic intraepithelial neoplasia and prostatic adenocarcinomas: A tissue microarray study. Journal of Clinical Pathology. 2011;**64**(8):683-688

[27] Miet SD, Neyra M, Jaques R, Dubernard P, Revol AA, Marçais MN, et al. RER+ phenotype in prostate intra-epithelial neoplasia associated with human prostate-carcinoma development. International Journal of Cancer. 1999;**82**(5):635-639

[28] Swinnen JV, Roskams T, Joniau S, Van Poppel H, Oyen R, Baert L, et al. Overexpression of fatty acid synthase is an early and common event in the development of prostate cancer. International Journal of Cancer. 2002;**98**(1):19-22

[29] Baltaci S, Orhan D, Özer G, Tolunay Ö, Gög? üs O. Bcl-2 proto-oncogene expression in low-and high-grade prostatic intraepithelial neoplasia. BJU International. 2000;**85**(1):155-159

[30] Qian J, Bostwick DG, Takahashi S, Borell TJ, Herath JF, Lieber MM, et al. Chromosomal anomalies in prostatic intraepithelial neoplasia and carcinoma detected by fluorescence in situ hybridization. Cancer Research. 1995;**55**(22):5408-5414

[31] Emmert-Buck MR, Vocke CD, Pozzatti RO, Duray PH, Jennings SB, Florence CD, et al. Allelic loss on chromosome 8p12-21 in microdissected prostatic intraepithelial neoplasia. Cancer Research. 1995;**55**(14):2959-2962

[32] Koeneman KS, Pan CX, Jin JK, Pyle JM, Flanigan RC, Shankey TV, et al. Telomerase activity, telomere length, and DNA ploidy in prostatic intraepithelial neoplasia (PIN). The Journal of Urology. 1998;**160**(4):1533-1539

[33] Brooks JD, Weinstein M, Lin X, Sun Y, Pin SS, Bova GS, et al. CG island methylation changes near the GSTP1 gene in prostatic intraepithelial neoplasia. Cancer Epidemiology, Biomarkers & Prevention: A Publication of the American Association for Cancer Research, Cosponsored by the American Society of Preventive Oncology. 1998;7(6):531-536

[34] Nakashiro KI, Hayashi Y, Oyasu R. Immunohistochemical expression of hepatocyte growth factor and c-met/HGF receptor in benign and malignant human prostate tissue. Oncology Reports. 2003;**10**(5):1149-1153

[35] Coogan CL, Bostwick DG, Bloom KJ, Gould VE. Glycoprotein A-80 in the human prostate: Immunolocalization in prostatic intraepithelial neoplasia, carcinoma, radiation failure, and after neoadjuvant hormonal therapy. Urology. 2003;**61**(1):248-252

[36] Hall RE, Horsfall DJ, Stahl J, Vivekanandan S, Ricciardelli C, Stapleton AM, et al. Apolipoprotein-D: A novel cellular marker for HGPIN and prostate cancer. The Prostate. 2004;**58**(2):103-108

[37] Henshall SM, Quinn DI, Lee CS, Head DR, Golovsky D, Brenner PC, et al. Overexpression of the cell cycle inhibitor p16INK4A in high-grade prostatic intraepithelial neoplasia predicts early relapse in prostate cancer patients. Clinical Cancer Research. 2001;**7**(3):544-550

[38] Hamilton W, Sharp DJ, Peters TJ, Round AP. Clinical features of prostate cancer before diagnosis: A population-based, case-control study. The British Journal of General Practice. 2006;**56**(531):756-762

[39] Reddy V, B, David O, Spitz DJ, Haber MH. Gattuso's Differential Diagnosis in Surgical Pathology. 4th ed. Philadelphia: Elsevier Health Sciences; 2021

[40] Fletcher CDM. Diagnostic Histopathology of Tumors, 2 Volume Set. 5th ed. Philadelphia: Elsevier; 2020

[41] Humphrey P. Variants of acinar adenocarcinoma of the prostate mimicking benign conditions. Modern Pathology. 2018;**31**(Suppl 1):64-70

[42] Warner JN, Nakamura LY, Pacelli A, Humphreys MR, Castle EP. Primary signet ring cell carcinoma of the prostate. Mayo Clinic Proceedings. 2010;**85**(12):1130-1136. DOI: 10.4065/mcp.2010.0463

[43] Bilé-Silva A, Lopez-Beltran A, Rasteiro H, Vau N, Blanca A, Gomez E,

et al. Pleomorphic giant cell carcinoma of the prostate: Clinicopathologic analysis and oncological outcomes. Virchows Archiv. 2023;**482**(3):493-505

[44] Paulk A, Giannico G, Epstein JI. PIN-like (ductal) adenocarcinoma of the prostate. The American Journal of Surgical Pathology. 2018;**42**(12):1693-1700. DOI: 10.1097/PAS.0000000000001139

[45] Epstein JI, Egevad L, Humphrey PA, et al. Best practices recommendations in the application of immuno-histochemistry in the prostate: Report from the International Society of Urologic Pathology consensus conference. The American Journal of Surgical Pathology. 2014;**38**(8):e6-e19

[46] Epstein JI, Egevad L, Humphrey PA, Montironi R, Members of the ISUP lmmunohistochemistry in Diagnostic Urologic Pathology Group. Best practices recommendations in the application of immunohistochemistry in lhe prostate: Report from the International Society of Urologic Pathology consensus conference. The American Journal of Surgical Pathology. 2014;**38**:e6-e19

[47] Hameed O, Humphrey PA. Lmmunohistochemistryin diagnostic surgical pathology of the prostate. Seminars in Diagnostic Pathology. 2005;**22**:88-104

[48] Brimo F, Epstein JI. Lmmuno-histochemicalpitfalls in prostate pathology. Human Pathology. 2012;**43**:313-324

[49] Jiang Z, Woda BA, Rock KL, et al. P504S: A new molecular marker for the detection of prostate carcinoma. The American Journal of Surgical Pathology. 2001;**25**(11):1397-1404

[50] Andrews C, Humphrey PA. Utility of ERG versus AMACR expression in diagnosis of minimal adenocarcinoma of the prostate in needle biopsy tissue. The American Journal of Surgical Pathology. 2014;**38**:1007-1012

[51] Gurel B, Ah TZ, Montgomery EA, Begum S, Hicks J, Goggins M, et al. NKX3.1 as a marker of prostatic origin in melaslalictumors. The American Journal of Surgical Pathology. 2010;**34**:1097-1105

[52] Varma M, Jasani B. Diagnostic utility of lrnrnunohislochemistry in morphologically difficult prostate cancer. Review of current literature. Histopathology. 2005;**47**:1-16

[53] Lane Z, Hansel DE, Epstein JI. Lmmunohistochemical expression of prostatic antigens in adenocarcinoma and villous adenoma of the urinary bladder. The American Journal of Surgical Pathology. 2008;**32**:322-326

[54] Cancer Genome Atlas Research Network. The molecular taxonomy of primary prostate cancer. Cell. 2015;**163**(4):1011-1025

[55] Armenia J, Wankowicz SAM, Liu D, et al. The long tail of oncogenic drivers in prostate cancer. Nature Genetics. 2018;**50**(5):645-651

[56] Arora K, Barbieri CE. Molecular subtypes of prostate cancer. Current Oncology Reports. 2018;**20**(8):58

[57] Robinson D, Van Allen EM, Wu YM, et al. Integrative clinical genomics of advanced prostate cancer. Cell. 2015;**162**(2):454

[58] Paulo P, Barras-Silva JD, Ribeiro FR, Ramalho-Carvalho J, Jerónimo C, Henrique R, et al. FLl 1 is a novel ETS transcription factor involved in gene fusions In prostate cancer. Genes, Chromosomes & Cancer. 2012;**51**:24-29

[59] Tomlins SA, Bjartell A, Chinnaiyan AM, Jenster G, Nam RK, Rubin MA, et al. ETS gene fusions in prostate cancer: From discovery to daily clinical practice. European Urology. 2009;**56**:275-286

[60] Taylor BS, Schultz N, Hieronymus H, et al. Integrative genomic profiling of human prostate cancer. Cancer Cell. 2010;**18**(1):11-22

[61] Hieronymus H, Schultz N, Gopalan A, et al. Copy number alteration burden predicts prostate cancer relapse. Proceedings of the National Academy of Sciences of the United States of America. 2014;**111**(30):11139-11144

[62] Li Y, Yang R, Henzler CM, et al. Diverse AR gene rearrangements mediate resistance to androgen receptor inhibitors in metastatic prostate cancer. Clinical Cancer Research. 2020;**26**(8):1965-1976

[63] Antonarakis ES, Lu C, Wang H, et al. AR-V7 and resistance to enzalutamide and abiraterone in prostate cancer. The New England Journal of Medicine. 2014;**371**(11):1028-1038

[64] Rescigno P, Gurel B, Pereira R, et al. Characterizing CDK12-mutated prostate cancers. Clinical Cancer Research. 2021;**27**(2):566-574

[65] Mateo J, Boysen G, Barbieri CE, et al. DNA repair in prostate cancer: Biology and clinical implications. European Urology. 2017;**71**(3):417-425

[66] Giri VN, Knudsen KE, Kelly WK, et al. Implementation of germline testing for prostate cancer: Philadelphia prostate cancer consensus conference 2019. Journal of Clinical Oncology. 2020;**38**(24):2798-2811

[67] Guedes LB, Antonarakis ES, Schweizer MT, et al. MSH2 loss in primary prostate cancer. Clinical Cancer Research. 2017;**23**(22):6863-6874

[68] Gleason DF. Histologic grading and clinical staging of prostate carcinoma. In: Tannenbaum M, editor. Urologic Pathology: The Prostate. Philadelphia: Lea & Febiger; 1977. pp. 171-198

[69] Epstein JI, Allsbrook WC Jr, Amin MB, et al. The 2005 International Society of Urological Pathology (ISUP) consensus conference on Gleason grading of prostatic carcinoma. The American Journal of Surgical Pathology. 2005;**29**(9):1228-1242

[70] Epstein JI, Egevad L, Amin MB, et al. The 2014 International Society of Urological Pathology (ISUP) consensus conference on Gleason grading of prostatic carcinoma: Definition of grading patterns and proposal for a new grading system. The American Journal of Surgical Pathology. 2016;**40**(2):244-252

[71] van Leenders GJLH, van der Kwast TH, Grignon DJ, et al. The 2019 International Society of Urological Pathology (ISUP) consensus conference on grading of prostatic carcinoma. The American Journal of Surgical Pathology. 2020;**44**(8):e87-e99

[72] Epstein JI, Amin MB, Fine SW, et al. The 2019 genitourinary pathology society (GUPS) white paper on contemporary grading of prostate cancer. Archives of Pathology & Laboratory Medicine. 2021;**145**(4):461-493

[73] Humphrey PA. Gleason grading and prognostic factors in carcinoma of the prostate. Modern Pathology. 2004;**17**:292-306

[74] Gaeta JF, Asirwatham JE, Miller G, et al. Histologic grading of primary prostatic cancer: A new approach to an

old problem. The Journal of Urology. 1980;**123**:689-693

[75] Amin MB, Grignon DJ, Humphrey PA, et al. Gleason Grading of Prostate Cancer: A Contemporary Approach. Philadelphia: Lippincott Williams and Wilkins; 2004. pp. 1-130

[76] Epstein JI, Amin MB, Reuter VE, et al. Contemporary Gleason grading of prostatic carcinoma: An update with discussion on practical issues to implement the 2014 International Society of Urological Pathology (ISUP) consensus conference on Gleason grading of prostatic carcinoma. The American Journal of Surgical Pathology. 2017;**41**(4):e1-e7

[77] Moch H, Humphrey PA, Ulbright TM, et al. WHO Classification of Tumours of the Urinary System and Male Genital Organs, WHO Classification of Tumours Series. 4th ed. Vol. 8. Lyon (France): International Agency for Research on Cancer; 2016. Available from: https://publications.iarc.fr/540

[78] Pierorazio PM, Walsh PC, Partin AW, et al. Prognostic Gleason grade grouping: Data based on the modified Gleason scoring system. BJU International. 2013;**111**(5):753-760

[79] Aus G, Damber JE, Khatami A, Lilja H, Stranne J, Hugosson J. Individualized screening interval for prostate cancer based on prostate-specific antigen level: Results of a prospective, randomized, population-based study. Archives of Internal Medicine. 2005;**165**(1):857-861

[80] Mistry K, Cable G. Meta-analysis of prostate-specific antigen and digital rectal examination as screening tests for prostate carcinoma. The Journal of the American Board of Family Practice. 2003;**16**:95-101

[81] Hernandez J, Thompson IM. Prostate-specific antigen: A review of the validation of the most commonly used cancer biomarker. Cancer. 2004;**101**:894-904

[82] Manna FL, Karkampouna S, Zoni E, et al. Metastases in prostate cancer. Cold Spring Harbor Perspectives in Medicine [Internet]. 2019;**9**(3):a033688

[83] Bubendorf L, Schöpfer A, Wagner U, et al. Metastatic patterns of prostate cancer: An autopsy study of 1,589 patients. Human Pathology. 2000;**31**(5):578-583

[84] American Cancer Society. Key statistics for prostate cancer. Prostate Cancer Facts [Internet]. 2024. Available from: https://www.cancer.org/cancer/types/prostate-cancer/about/key-statistics.html

[85] Buhmeida A, Pyrhönen S, Laato M, Collan Y. Prognostic factors in prostate cancer. Diagnostic Pathology. 2006;**1**(4):1-15

[86] Martin NE, Mucci LA, Loda M, Depinho RA. Prognostic determinants in prostate cancer. Cancer Journal. 2011;**17**(6):429-437

[87] Paner GP, Srigley JR, Pettus J, et al. Protocol for the Examination of Radical Prostatectomy Specimens from Patients with Carcinoma of the Prostate Gland. USA: College of American Pathologists [Internet]; 2021

[88] Mott LM. Squamous cell carcinoma of the prostate: Report of 2 cases and review of the literature. The Journal of Urology. 1979;**121**(6):833-835

[89] Nabi G, Ansari MS, Singh I, Sharma MC, Dogra PN. Primary squamous cell carcinoma of the prostate: A rare clinicopathological entity: Report of 2 cases and review of literature. Urologia. 2001;**66**(4):216-219

[90] Hanna K, Lele SM, McCormick G, McMahon A, Hill B, Boyle SL. Primary prostatic squamous cell carcinoma. Urology Case Reports. 2021;**34**:101478

[91] Malik RD, Dakwar G, Hardee ME, Sanfilippo NJ, Rosenkrantz AB, Taneja SS. Squamous cell carcinoma of the prostate. Reviews in Urology. 2011;**13**(1):56

[92] Biswas T, Podder T, Lepera PA, Walker P. Primary squamous cell carcinoma of the prostate: A case report of a rare clinical entity. Future Science OA. 2015;**1**(3):FSO18

[93] Sieracki JC. Epidermoid carcinoma of the human prostate: Report of three cases. Laboratory Investigation; A Journal of Technical Methods and Pathology. 1955;**4**(3):232-240

[94] Kahler JE. Carcinoma of the prostate gland: A pathologic study. The Journal of Urology. 1939;**41**(4):557-574

[95] Bennett RS, Edgertont EO. Mixed prostatic carcinoma. The Journal of Urology. 1973;**110**(5):561-563

[96] Gattuso P, Carson HJ, Candel A, Castelli MJ. Adenosquamous carcinoma of the prostate. Human Pathology. 1995;**26**(1):123-126

[97] Devaney DM, Dorman A, Leader M. Adenosquamous carcinoma of the prostate: A case report. Human Pathology. 1991;**22**(10):1046-1050

[98] Moyana TN. Adenosquamous carcinoma of the prostate. The American Journal of Surgical Pathology. 1987;**11**(5):403-407

[99] Ulloa SA, Iturregui JR, Amezquita M, Ortiz VN. Squamous cell carcinoma of the prostate: Case report and review of literature. Boletin de la Asociacion Medica de Puerto Rico. 1997;**89**(10-12):192-194

[100] Lager DJ, Goeken JA, Kemp JD, Robinson RA. Squamous metaplasia of the prostate: An immunohistochemical study. American Journal of Clinical Pathology. 1988;**90**(5):597-601

[101] Munoz F, Franco P, Ciammella P, Clerico M, Giudici M, Filippi AR, et al. Squamous cell carcinoma of the prostate: Long-term survival after combined chemo-radiation. Radiation Oncology. 2007;**2**:1-7

[102] Brunnhoelzl D, Wang J. Clinical features, treatment, prognosis, and outcome of 47 patients with pure squamous cell carcinoma of the prostate. Journal of Clinical Oncology. 2018;**36**:7

[103] Mishra S, Goel H, Awasthi N, Puri A, Mahapatra R, Pal DK. Primary adenosquamous carcinoma of the prostate: A rare aggressive tumor. Clinical Genitourinary Cancer. 2014;**12**(1):e29-e31

[104] Parwani AV, Kronz JD, Genega EM, Gaudin P, Chang S, Epstein JI. Prostate carcinoma with squamous differentiation: An analysis of 33 cases. The American Journal of Surgical Pathology. 2004;**28**(5):651-657

[105] Bassler TJ Jr, Orozco R, Bassler IC, Boyle LM, Bormes T. Adenosquamous carcinoma of the prostate: Case report with DNA analysis, immunohistochemistry, and literature review. Urology. 1999;**53**(4):832-834

[106] Kin T, Tsukamoto T, Yonese J, Ishikawa Y, Fukui I. Adenosquamous carcinoma of the prostate with elevated serum parathyroid hormonerelatedprotein and squamous cell carcinoma antigen. BJU International. 2000;**86**(4):562

[107] Orhan D, Dizbay Sak S, Yaman Ö, Tulunay Ö, Gög˘üş O. Adenosquamous carcinoma of the prostate. British Journal of Urology. 1996;**78**(4):646-647

[108] Hennessey A, Buller D, Sama S, Girard E, Clement J, Ristau BT. Case report: Adenosquamous carcinoma of the prostate with greater than 20 month response to multimodal therapy. Urology Case Reports. 2020;**29**:101084

[109] Riegman PH, Oomen MH, Dinjens WN, Oosterhuis JW, Lam KH, Spatz A, et al. TuBaFrost: European virtual tumor tissue banking. Advances in Experimental Medicine and Biology. 2006;**587**:65-74

[110] Su X, Long Q, Bo J, Shi Y, Zhao LN, Lin Y, et al. Mutational and transcriptomic landscapes of a rare human prostate basal cell carcinoma. The Prostate. 2020;**80**(6):508-517

[111] Dong S, Liu Q, Xu Z, Wang H. An unusual case of metastatic basal cell carcinoma of the prostate: A case report and literature review. Frontiers in Oncology. 2020;**27**(10):859

[112] Ayyathurai R, Civantos F, Soloway MS, Manoharan M. Basal cell carcinoma of the prostate: Current concepts. BJU International. 2007;**99**(6):1345-1349

[113] Minei S, Hachiya T, Ishida H, Okada K. Adenoid cystic carcinoma of the prostate: A case report with immunohistochemical and in situ hybridization staining for prostate-specific antigen. International Journal of Urology. 2001;**8**(8):S41-S44

[114] Epstein JI, Netto GJ. Prostate and seminal vesicles. In: Mills and Sternberg's Diagnostic Surgical Pathology. 6th ed. Philadelphia, Pennsylvania: Wolters Kluwer; 2022

[115] Zhou M, Tavora F, Pan C, et al. Prostatic stromal tumour of uncertain malignant potential. In: WHO Classification of Tumours Editorial Board, editor. Urinary and Male Genital Tumours [Internet], WHO Classification of Tumours Series. 5th ed. Vol. 8. Lyon (France): International Agency for Research on Cancer; 2022

Section 2

Innovations in Management of Benign Prostatic Hyperplasia

Chapter 3

Anatomical Endoscopic Enucleation of the Prostate: An Overview

Ajay Bhandarkar, Nisarg Mehta and Rishabh Handa

Abstract

Lower urinary tract symptoms (LUTS) increase with age, primarily due to benign prostatic obstruction (BPO), affecting about 80% of men above 80 years of age with a significant impact on quality of life (QoL). Treatment varies from pharmacotherapy to surgery based on the severity of LUTS. Transurethral resection of prostate (TURP) has been considered the standard of care for surgical management of LUTS/BPO. However, in the last few decades with technological advancements and shortfalls of TURP, newer techniques for surgical treatment have emerged. These techniques score over TURP in many ways providing significant functional improvements, shorter hospital stays, and lower complication rates compared to conventional resection techniques. Advancements in laser technology and surgical approaches have established anatomical endoscopic enucleation of the prostate (AEEP) as a gold standard for benign prostatic hyperplasia (BPH) surgery. AEEP offers excellent functional outcomes, reduced bleeding risks, shorter catheterization times, and lower hospital stays, making it suitable for a wide range of patients, especially those with large prostates. Long-term functional outcomes of AEEP are superior to TURP irrespective of the technique or energies used. Future research should aim to optimize surgical techniques, explore ejaculatory-sparing approaches, and standardize outcome reporting to further solidify AEEP's role in BPO treatment.

Keywords: benign prostatic hyperplasia, laser enucleation of the prostate, benign prostatic obstruction, holmium laser, lower urinary tract symptoms, surgical intervention

1. Introduction

The prevalence of LUTS increases with age, and it is predominantly due to BPH in men, which ultimately impairs QoL [1, 2]. Approximately 80% of men over the age of 80 years old experience LUTS. LUTS interfere with daily functioning, and elderly males with LUTS often feel emotional discomfort, such as depressive mood and anxiety [3]. The severity of LUTS and the risk of progression determines the choice of therapy in BPH. Pharmacotherapy for BPH has shown a morbidity of >10% in one of the reported studies [4]. Indications for the surgery include failure of medical therapy to reduce bothersome LUTS, intolerable pharmaceutical side effects, or the desire by

IntechOpen

the patient to avoid taking long-term medical management. Other absolute indications for the surgical treatment are acute and/or chronic renal insufficiency, refractory urinary retention, recurrent urinary tract infections (UTIs), recurrent bladder stones, and recalcitrant gross hematuria [5].

Removal of the obstructing prostatic adenoma by open surgical enucleation, open prostatectomy (OP), is the oldest surgical treatment modality for moderate-to-severe LUTS secondary to BPH. OP reduces LUTS by 63–86%, improves IPSS-QoL score by 60–87%, and increases maximum flow rate (Qmax) by 375% with a reduction of post-void residue (PVR) by 86–98% [6]. Despite excellent clinical outcomes and long-term efficacy, several decades ago, OP was replaced by TURP. It was due to advancements in endoscopic equipment and reduced peri-operative morbidity following transurethral resection. TURP is still regarded as the standard surgical procedure for the treatment of LUTS secondary to BPO in small to medium (30-80 grams) prostates. No studies on the optimal cut-off value exist, but the complication rates after TURP increase with prostate size [7]. Transurethral (TUR) syndrome, bleeding, and infectious complications in the perioperative period following monopolar TURP (M-TURP) were the main reason to look for alternate sources of energy to be used in transurethral procedures which can be equally efficacious with minimum morbidity [8]. Bipolar TURP (B-TURP) has similar efficacy as compared to M-TURP but with lower peri-operative morbidity. Long-term results (up to 5 years) for B-TURP showed that safety and efficacy are comparable to M-TURP [9].

Newer minimally invasive surgical treatment options for BPH have developed in the last three decades. Holmium laser enucleation of the prostate (HoLEP) was introduced in 1998 [10] marking the beginning of interest in endoscopic enucleation for the treatment of BPH. HoLEP proved to be safe and effective, especially in large prostates in many studies [11, 12]. Even non-laser energy like bipolar electrocautery, which was being used for the resection of prostatic adenoma, was found to be effective in the endoscopic enucleation of the prostate [13]. Laser energies like thulium yttrium-aluminum-garnet (YAG), potassium-titanyl-phosphate (KTP), and diode were initially used for vaporization or resection of the prostatic adenoma. The use of end-firing fibers in thulium/diode/greenlight lasers and concepts of separating prostate adenoma from the capsule in the proper surgical plane for enucleation established the fact that the technique of enucleation was more important than the energy used for enucleation [14]. The acronym anatomical endoscopic enucleation of the prostate (AEEP) was coined by Hermann in his editorial [15]. It became "standard of care" in the surgical treatment of BPH once it was included as a treatment of choice in many guidelines [16]. The major advantage of AEEP is the ability to remove the adenoma close to the anatomical plane between the surgical capsule and the adenoma. It is similar to what the index finger does during an OP procedure making it equally efficacious. Several studies demonstrated no significant differences between AEEP and OP in short and intermediate-term functional outcomes. The requirement of blood transfusion was significantly less with AEEP compared to OP [17, 18].

The overall morbidity of TURP is not statistically significant compared to minimally invasive treatment modalities, but the possibility of TUR syndrome is higher with M-TURP. The diversity of possible complications after TURP leads to an increased cumulative risk of adverse events. According to a meta-analysis published in 2010 [19], the most relevant complications include bleeding requiring blood transfusion (2%; range: 0–9), TUR syndrome (0.8%; range: 0–5), acute urinary retention (AUR) (4.5%; range: 0–13.3), clot retention (4.9%; range: 0–39), and UTI (4.1%; range: 0–22). However, the size of the prostate and surgical experience plays a major role in TURP-related complications.

Endoscopic enucleation of the prostate (EEP) procedures remove a maximum amount of prostatic tissue, which is equivalent to open enucleation leading to complete resolution of obstruction. Enucleation is beneficial compared to resection in reducing hospital stay, hemoglobin loss, serum sodium decrease, blood transfusion rate, grade II, grade III complications, and early postoperative complications [20]. A study published by Madersbacher et al. [21] in 2005 reported a cumulative incidence of secondary TURP procedures of 2.9, 5.8, and 7.4% at 1, 5, and 8 years, respectively, following the procedure. HoLEP is the most widely analyzed and reported endoscopic enucleation procedure. The risk of re-operation following HoLEP was variable in different published studies [21]. An interesting meta-analysis [22] published in 2020 reported that there was no statistical difference in functional outcomes following the use of laser or non-laser energy sources for EEP. However, the overall weight of the prostatic tissue enucleated was higher (no clinical significance) and hemoglobin drop was lower when laser energy source was used.

The surgical treatment for LUTS seems to be safe for all age groups as the mortality after any transurethral procedures was found to be less than 0.5%. AEEP has marginally less mortality compared to TURP. Higher postoperative mortality is believed to be associated with increasing age, high Charlson Comorbidity Index (CCI) score, and atrial fibrillation as independent risk factors [23]. It is strongly recommended to carefully consider the type of surgical procedure and weigh the risks and benefits on a case-to-case basis.

2. The evolution of AEEP

Many medical technologies have evolved because of cumulative selection, and EEP is no exception. TURP has been the gold standard surgical treatment for BPH for decades. However, the morbidities following TURP, such as risk of TUR syndrome, bleeding complications, and limitations of resection for large prostate size (>100 grams), were the driving factors to shift to EEP. The first transurethral prostate enucleation was reported by Hiraoka and Akimoto in 1989 [24]. They reported a case series of 200 patients in which a bespoke blade was used to detach the adenoma from the prostate capsule.

A feasible transurethral endoscopic enucleation procedure could once again become a possibility with the advancement and application of laser technology in urology. Gilling and Fraundorfer [25] developed the HoLEP technique in Tauranga, New Zealand, in the mid-1990s. The evolution of this technique which started as an ablative procedure to the current enucleation one is due to the advances in the morcellation techniques and laser technology. Before holmium laser, neodymium: Yttrium-aluminum-garnet (Nd: YAG) laser was used for vapo-laser ablation of prostate (VLAP). It did not gain much enthusiasm due to concerns like delayed time to voiding and post-surgery dysuria. To overcome these shortfalls, Gilling et al. in 1994 introduced hybrid/combination endoscopic laser ablation of the prostate (CELAP) technique using the Nd:YAG laser for circumferential coagulation followed by holmium laser ablation. Thus, a 60-watt laser with a single-use, side-firing fiber was used to vaporize the prostate's surface in the first pure holmium-only laser ablation of the prostate (HoLAP) in 1994 [25]. The advantages of this procedure were good hemostasis, short hospital stays, and an easy learning curve; however, cons included longer operative times, higher cost, and no tissue available for histopathology. To minimize the cost, Gilling et al. introduced reusable end firing fibers and used them to resect the prostate; hence, the technique of Holmium Laser resection of prostate (HoLRP) was developed. During this evolving process, it was also realized conceptually that a plane between the prostate adenoma and the prostate capsule could be created endoscopically with ease, much like a surgeon's finger shelling out an adenoma during an open retropubic prostatectomy. Hence, the term HoLEP was coined. Four key steps of HoLEP included: (1) creation of bladder neck incisions, (2) enucleation of the median lobe, (3) enucleation of the lateral lobes, and (4) transurethral morcellation. Initial results showed equivalent outcomes as compared to TURP and better feasibility in larger prostates (>100 g). Many improvements for tissue morcellators developed leading to increased acceptability of this technique among urologists. Various modifications in the way enucleation was done have been described in the literature, for example, mushroom technique, en-bloc enucleation with all achieving the same overall results [13, 26].

Different energy sources were used following the same principles of HoLEP. In early 2000s, bipolar electrocautery was used for vaporization of prostate tissue. In 2006, Neil et al. [13] presented a randomized control trial between HoLEP and plasmakinetic bipolar enucleation of the prostate, which was found to be feasible with similar outcomes. The popularity of transurethral enucleation of the prostate using bipolar energy (TUEB) grew in Asia (especially China), and various modifications in the technique and instruments evolved over time. Liu et al. [27] published their study of transurethral enucleation and resection of the prostate (TUERP) with plasmakinetic energy in 2010. He popularized the concept of using mechanical energy (tip of the resectoscope) for the enucleation of adenoma in proper anatomical plane, coagulating the feeding blood vessels and creating large, detached adenomas which were attached to the prostatic fossa at the bladder neck. These almost avascular adenomas were then resected with the bipolar electrocautery to complete the procedure. The aim of the procedure was to use single set of instruments to do the entire job, avoid morcellation procedure, and hence reduce the cost of treatment. Transurethral enucleation with bipolar (TUEB) using the transurethral resection in saline (TURis) system (Olympus) and the TUEB loop was developed by Olympus Corporation (Tokyo, Japan). Ken Nakagawa introduced the TUEB technique, by using the novel TUEB loop [28]. This bipolar electrocautery loop with enucleating spatula was useful for resection and enucleation with normal saline as irrigation. TUEB results were better than standard TURis technique, especially in large prostates. The 'button' type vapo-resection electrode (Olympus Europe, Hamburg, Germany) was designed to use for vaporization of the prostate. But it was soon realized that, the button has enough strength to be used for mechanical enucleation of the adenoma off the capsule. The plasma-button enucleation technique, termed as bipolar enucleation of the prostate (BPEP), was reported to have significantly lower peri-operative morbidity and an improved post-operative recovery when compared with standard OP [29].

In 2005, Xia et al. [30] were the first to describe a technique using the thulium laser for resection of the prostate, whereby the prostate was cut into slices in what they termed the 'tangerine technique'. Bach and Hermann et al. [31] described the vapo-resection of prostate in 2005, using the thulium laser system. In 2010, Herrmann et al. [32] described the three-lobe technique for thulium laser enucleation of the prostate (ThuLEP) with comparable functional results as HoLEP.

Greenlight laser prostate surgery was first described with a so-called, photo-vaporization of prostate (PVP) technique [33]. One of the limitations of PVP is the challenge encountered in large-volume prostates (>90 ml) in completely vaporizing the transitional zone. With PVP, operating times are longer, and retreatment rates can be as high as 9%. In 2015, Gomez Sancha et al. [34] described greenlight laser enucleation of the prostate (GreenLEP) to overcome these problems. It involved logical steps from standard vaporization to anatomic vaporization, then to vapo-enucleation, and finally to en-bloc enucleation. GreenLEP is a newer enucleation technique, and there is still a paucity of data concerning the long-term effectiveness of this approach.

The 982 nm wavelength high power diode laser was introduced in 2009 for rapid ablation of the prostate tissue [35]. The Eraser laser with a 1318 nm diode laser was found to be effective for cutting, coagulating, and sealing. It was compared with high-power PVP laser for ablation. Lusardi et al. [36] explored the use of this laser for prostate enucleation and reported it to be safe and effective for EEP. Diode laser enucleation of the prostate (DiLEP) for the treatment of BPH when compared with bipolar enucleation was non-inferior at one-year follow-up [37, 38].

The technique of AEEP has evolved over the last two decades. There is more than enough evidence to support its efficacy and safety in the surgical treatment of BPH.

3. Why choose AEEP over TURP?

TURP has remained 'the gold standard' in the surgical management of benign prostatic enlargement (BPE) for decades. Many different modalities for the surgical management for BPE have been suggested in recent times. AEEP has stood out as one of the best options for many reasons. It primarily differs from TURP in that the entire adenomatous tissue is removed.

During TURP, one encounters bleeding vessels in most of the swipes as one resects through the adenomatous tissue, whereas in AEEP, blood vessels are encountered only on the inner surface of the peripheral zone as they perforate into the transitional zone. In a meta-analysis done by Wroclawski et al. in 2020, it was concluded that there was a statistically significant difference with reduced drop in hemoglobin, a lesser requirement of blood transfusions, shorter catheter time, shorter hospital stay in AEEP as compared to resection techniques [22].

One of the most important and widely accepted advantages of AEEP is in large prostates. The larger the prostate, the portion of the transitional zone (TZ) removed may be smaller, and the inter-surgeon variability in terms of completeness of adenoma removal is greater in TURP. Therefore, outcomes for vaporization and resection are less good for men with larger prostates. Kuntz et al. [39] reported that surgical re-treatment rates were significantly higher in TURP than those reported for AEEP in men with large prostates at 5-year follow-up. Gilling et al. [40] followed patients in their randomized trial comparing HoLEP versus TURP to a mean of 7.6 years. None in the HoLEP group had required a re-operation compared to 18% in the TURP group. A meta-analysis by Morozov et al. [41] done in 2023 showed that AEEP had a significantly lower re-operation rate and better functional outcomes (Qmax and IPSS) in long term compared with TURP. It may also be beneficial in terms of the International Index for Erectile Function (IIEF-5), PVR, and Prostate Specific Antigen (PSA) levels. Hence, it offers better safety and efficacy for a wider range of patients than any other procedure for prostatic enlargement.

4. The technique of AEEP

In AEEP, removal of the prostate adenoma is done by following a natural anatomical plane. In theory, this procedure when done properly, should be able to achieve maximal efficacy in a minimally invasive manner. Fraundorfer et al. [10] exploited this plane to launch HoLEP in 1998. It was following the same principles of OP carried out by the transurethral route. However, longer operative time, steep learning curve, and fear of urinary incontinence compelled further studies to modify the technique of enucleation. Several investigators used different energy sources (thulium/diode/greenlight lasers, bipolar electrocautery) following the same surgical steps for AEEP.

1. *"Three-lobe technique"* where two longitudinal incisions from the bladder neck to verumontanum at 5 and 7 o'clock positions are made initially. These two incisions are joined proximal to verumontanum, and the entire median lobe is enucleated in a retrograde manner. Two lateral lobes are then enucleated after separating them by a third longitudinal incision at 12 o'clock position and two vertical incisions distally around the apical region to separate the adenoma from its capsule proximal to the sphincter zone muscle fibers. Three lobes of prostatic adenoma enucleated independently from the prostatic fossa and pushed into the urinary bladder for removal by morcellation [10, 40]. Subsequently, many studies tried to simplify the technique by offering some modifications. Hochreiter [26] described a "mushroom technique" whereby the enucleated prostate adenoma was kept attached to the prostate fossa at the bladder neck which was later resected with electrocautery to avoid a morcellation procedure.

2. *"Two-lobe technique"* published by Dusing et al. [42] reported that enucleation efficiency can be improved with modification of the technique and experience. A solitary posterior groove is made, and the median lobe is included in the enucleation of one of the lateral lobes, which saves operative time in large prostates. They also advocated the initiation of enucleation at the apex lateral to the verumontanum, as opposed to 12 o'clock anterior, as the plane between the adenoma and capsule is easy to identify around the verumontanum. Dissection is then carried lateral and circumferential to separate the lateral lobes. An early apical release by incising mucosa over the apical region and avoiding stress and strain of mechanical manipulations on the sphincter zone was found to reduce the incidences of urinary incontinence (UI) following this technique.

3. *"En-bloc technique"* is the modification where all three lobes of the prostate are enucleated as one unit. Enucleation is begun by incising mucosa around verumontanum and defining the posterior capsule. Then, the surgical plane is widened circumferentially and in retrograde fashion from the apical region to the bladder neck. Many variants of "en-bloc" enucleation are reported by different investigators [43, 44] claiming the superiority of their techniques. The '*en-bloc*' techniques with early apical liberation have emerged with many theoretical advantages: better visualization, faster identification of the surgical capsule and the correct plane to dissect reduced operating time and amount of energy delivered, better preservation of the sphincter, and an improved learning curve compared to the three-lobe technique [45, 46].

Future larger comparative studies are needed to evaluate true impact of the technique on outcomes of AEEP.

5. Energies used for the AEEP

After Fraundorfer et al. [10] described the possibility of EEP with the use of holmium laser in 1998, many researchers tried to use various energy sources for EEP to match the results of HoLEP or improve it further. Much cited editorial [15] by Herrmann in 2016 steered discussion on focusing AEEP as a new gold standard surgical treatment in the BPO. Maximum studies comparing outcomes and complications among all AEEP techniques have been done with HoLEP; on the other hand, GreenLEP is the least studied one. It was soon realized that anatomical knowledge and the technique of enucleation were more important than the energies used for enucleation.

1. *The holmium laser* has a wavelength of roughly 2140 nm and can penetrate tissue for 0.4 to 0.5 mm. Holmium lasers operate in a pulsed form. High peak pressures have more mechanical effects on the tissues compared to thulium laser. This helps the holmium laser to follow the path of least resistance between the adenoma and the surgical capsule. That may be the reason, HoLEP is considered to be more anatomic. However, many meta-analyses and studies found no significant differences in peri-operative or functional parameters [47].

2. *The Thulium: YAG laser* transmits energy as a continuous wave with a wavelength close to 2000 nm and its increased affinity for water absorption makes it an excellent vaporizing and cutting laser. ThuLEP uses blunt dissection to a greater extent and laser energy is used as and when it is necessary. The cutting ability of ThuLEP may be beneficial in some situations, as anatomical enucleation is not necessarily required. With the whole range of surgical approaches for transurethral prostatectomy for BPO, including vaporization, resection, enucleation, and vapo-enucleation, thulium:YAG offers the best choice.

3. *The diode laser* has the strongest tissue penetration capabilities with an effective distance of 5 mm. Its capacity to harm the surgical capsule of the prostate when used for prostate enucleation cannot be disregarded [48]. The diode lasers have the physical properties of a high energy conversion efficiency. Small and portable size of the machine may contribute as favorable factors in their use for clinical practice. The literature lacks robust studies showing comparison of diode laser use for EEP with other widely used lasers like holmium and thulium.

4. *The greenlight laser* is one of the lasers with good tissue penetration performance, according to an investigation of physical parameters. The thermodynamic conduction distance is 1–2 mm, and its optical visible penetrating ability is 0.8–0.9 mm. At the same time, it works in the continuous mode. Although the mechanical effect can be avoided, the tissue damage caused by the thermodynamic effect of the continuous working mode, and the strong tissue penetration is worthy of attention [34].

5. *Bipolar* endoscopic enucleation of the prostate (BEEP) includes a large range of procedures, such as plasmakinetic enucleation of the prostate (PkEP), transurethral resection enucleation of the prostate (TUERP), bipolar plasma enucleation of the prostate (BPEP), transurethral vapor-enucleation resection of the prostate (TVERP), transurethral vapor-enucleation of the prostate (TVEP) and, finally, bipolar enucleation of the prostate (BipoLEP). All enucleation procedures with bipolar energy have found to be better than bipolar TURP in terms of efficacy and safety. Many studies have reported bipolar enucleation of the prostate as a safer alternative with equally comparable outcomes with OP or HoLEP [49].

6. *The thulium fiber laser (TFL)* is an advanced tool suitable for both soft tissue procedures and lithotripsy, utilizing two operational modes: quasi-continuous wave (QCW) and super pulsed (SP). The QCW mode, similar to the thulium:YAG laser, is specifically used for soft tissue surgeries such as the surgical treatment of BPH or non-muscle invasive bladder cancer (NMIBC). The SP mode, akin to the Holmium:YAG laser, applies to both soft tissue and stone surgeries [50]. TFL has a wavelength of 1940 nm with a maximum water absorption peak in tissue. It has a theoretical tissue penetration depth of 100 micron. Since soft tissues are predominantly composed of water (*80%), the thermal effects of TFL make it more precise for cutting compared to holmium laser. Key distinctions between SP TFL and Ho:YAG include SP TFL's higher potential frequency (up to 2000 Hz compared to Ho: YAG's 50-80 Hz), lower peak power (500 W for SP TFL vs. 2-10 kW for Ho: YAG), and longer pulse duration (500 milliseconds for TFL vs. 350 milliseconds for Ho: YAG) [51]. The area of coagulation with holmium laser is larger compared to TFL, so no carbonization is seen with holmium laser. TFL appears to be an efficient alternative to Ho:YAG laser for soft tissue surgery. TFL not only boasts beneficial properties for surgical procedures but also offers enhanced usability and serviceability [52]. Its setup is more compact and lighter than the Ho: YAG systems, requiring less space in the operating theater and easing its use. TFL operates on standard 220 V or 110 V electrical sockets, simplifying installation requirements in smaller surgical spaces. Additionally, TFL is quieter during operation, as noted by Moore et al., improving communication among surgical staff during procedures and enhancing the overall comfort for surgeons and nurses [53].

Holmium laser has stood the test of time; it has been extensively studied and has become the gold standard for laser prostatectomy. A contemporary sophistication of the holmium laser has been the development of pulse modulation, in which two consecutive rapid pulses are emitted [54]. This Moses Technology makes it possible to preserve dissection properties and also offers improved cutting plus coagulative effect.

Recent advancements in both thulium and holmium lasers with pulse modulation capacity are a significant leap forward for the safe and efficient AEEP. It is a matter of personal preference regarding which energy source is better for EEP.

6. Learning curve for AEEP

EEP is generally considered more challenging to learn than TURP due to the need for precise identification of the correct tissue layer. Various methods, including step-by-step techniques and newer, potentially simpler approaches, have been proposed to reduce the EEP learning curve. Herrmann [14] noted that prostate enucleation offers consistent efficacy and safety across different energy sources, though no similar claim has been made regarding ease of learning. The learning curve's length can vary significantly, requiring between 15 and 80 procedures to master [55, 56]. A systematic review done by Kampantais et al. [57] highlighted the critical nature of this learning curve, showing that initial training phases could lead to more frequent relapses and complications, as evidenced by their review of 24 studies on HoLEP.

Mastering HoLEP typically requires performing 30-40 cases, with proficiency plateauing after 20 to 60 cases, though certain efficiencies continue to improve [58]. Lerner et al. [59] found that extended intervals between procedures (over 5 weeks) significantly raise the risk of incontinence, underscoring the need for consistent practice to minimize complications.

A study by Peyronnet et al. [60] comparing GreenLEP and HoLEP found a slightly quicker learning curve for GreenLEP in achieving operative benchmarks, with complication rates stabilizing after 30 cases for HoLEP but remaining consistently low for GreenLEP. ThuLEP and ThuFLEP have learning curves of about 30 and 20 cases, respectively, while TUEB requires 40–50 cases to master [61]. Enikeev et al. noted that methods using electric energy are more challenging to learn than laser techniques, although no specific case number was provided [62, 63]. Xiong et al. observed that inexperienced surgeons might switch from TUEB to bipolar resection in challenging cases, opting to manually cut tissue instead of using morcellation upon enucleation completion [64].

EEP learning curve assessment is varied, often showing a diminishing return pattern as many surgeons have prior endourology experience. While early progress is described as "steep," implying rapid learning, the term lacks a strict definition. Complication rates and the number of procedures (ranging from 20 to 200 for proficiency) are influenced by the surgeon's prior experience and the time between cases.

7. Complications of AEEP

AEEP is likely to become a "future standard" in the surgical treatment of BPH. However, peri-operative complications of AEEP are inevitable although the incidence is reducing with refinements of the technique.

Transient urinary incontinence (UI) is a common complication after AEEP, but most patients recover within 3–6 months. The incidence of UI is significantly related to the surgeon's experience [65]. It was reported that approximately 16.6–29.4% of patients suffered from post-operative UI within 6 months after HoLEP, but only 0–3.3% of patients could not recover automatically at 12 months [66]. Krambeck et al. [67] reported that at short-term, intermediate term, long-term, and greater than 5-year follow-up, stress incontinence was noted in 12.5, 3.4, 1.8, and 4.8% of patients, respectively. The incidence of UI after BipoLEP was 6.8%, among which 91.3% of patients recovered 3 months after surgery and 97.5% of patients recovered 6 months after surgery. Age $\geq$ 70 years and prostate volume $\geq$ 90 mL were associated with post-operative SUI [68]. The number of previous surgical cases is a predictor of transient UI, with a higher number of cases associated with a lower incidence of incontinence. Other factors that can predict post-operative incontinence include the IPSS, pre-operative detrusor overactivity (DO), patient's age, and surgeon mentorship [69].

The overall incidence of peri-operative hemorrhage requiring blood transfusions after AEEP is approximately 1.2-1.9% of BPO patients [70, 71]. Mean hemoglobin before and after HoLEP decreased from 14.6 to 12.3 g/dl, and mean hematocrit decreased from 44.3 to 37.7% [72].

Adverse events after HoLEP are considered quite rare, and most complications develop early during the surgeon learning curve, emphasizing the importance of the mentorship process in improving the surgeon learning curve and reducing potential complications. For instance, the risk of bleeding and blood transfusion is lower for HoLEP than for TURP and open prostatectomy. The transfusion rate of 0.8% reinforces the safety of this procedure even in anticoagulated cases [72].

A bladder neck contracture is another complication of AEEP, with a high recurrence rate. It occurs in about 0.8% of patients undergoing AEEP [73]. The incidence of bladder neck contracture is comparable between different AEEP techniques, such as HoLEP, BipoLEP, ThuLEP, and GreenLEP. The main cause of postoperative bladder neck contracture is mechanical and thermal impairment to the bladder neck during surgery. Other risk factors for bladder neck contracture include pre-operative urinary tract infections, excessive diameter of the device, and prolonged post-operative catheterization. Techniques that preserve the prostatic apex or reduce the tension in the external sphincter can help reduce the incidence of bladder neck contracture as well as maintain ejaculatory function.

With an incidence of 1.2–7.3%, urethral stricture is a complication that can occur after various types of prostatectomies [72, 73]. The incidence of urethral stricture after AEEP is significantly lower compared to TURP and open surgery [72]. However, the incidence of urethral stricture is similar between AEEP techniques such as HoLEP, ThuLEP, and DiLEP [14]. Risk factors for urethral stricture include mechanical impairment, intra-operative incision due to the confined urethral meatus, urinary tract infection, and prolonged catheterization. Pre-operative urethral dilation increased lubricant use, and shortened operation time can help reduce the occurrence of urethral stricture [12].

Sexual dysfunction is another important consideration in BPH surgery. Retrograde ejaculation is the most common sexual dysfunction after AEEP, with a high incidence (>75%). The incidence of retrograde ejaculation is similar between AEEP and TURP [74]. Preserving the bladder neck during surgery may help reduce the occurrence of retrograde ejaculation, but the impact of bladder neck preservation on ejaculation remains controversial. Erectile dysfunction is rarely observed after AEEP. ThuLEP has been shown to have a minimal effect on erectile function, and the power intensity used in HoLEP does not affect erectile function [75].

In conclusion, AEEP is a safe surgical procedure for the treatment of BPH with lower complication rates compared to open surgery and TURP. Transient UI is a common complication, but most patients recover within a few months. Bladder neck contracture and urethral stricture are more serious complications that require further research to develop prevention and treatment strategies. Retrograde ejaculation is a common sexual dysfunction after AEEP, but erectile function is generally preserved. Surgeon experience and technique play a significant role in reducing the incidence of complications.

8. Functional outcomes of AEEP

AEEP is considered technically challenging when compared with TURP. All guidelines outline that it is the experience of the surgeon that has the largest impact on complications and clinical outcomes. Maximum studies comparing outcomes and complications among all AEEP techniques have been done with HoLEP, and on the other hand, GreenLEP is the least studied one. The key outcomes – IPSS,

Qmax, reduction in PVR, operation time and complications – were routinely utilized as essential indicators for assessing the surgical therapy of BPH in majority of the studies.

European Association of Urology (EAU) guidelines summary published in 2024 strongly recommends Holmium YAG laser enucleation for large prostates only [76]. Recommendation is weak for thulium YAG laser, and there is insufficient evidence for all other laser-based procedures. Yucheng Ma et al. studied various enucleation techniques by a network meta-analysis (NMA) method [77]. They reported that diode lasers did not exhibit statistically significant advantages or drawbacks over other types of lasers in terms of safety and efficacy. Greenlight laser demonstrated the weakest performance according to this NMA study.

In a prospective and randomized trial with 133 patients, Zhang et al. reported that ThuLEP required longer operation time (72.6 vs. 61.5 min) but resulted in less blood loss compared to HoLEP [78]. However, many meta-analyses reported no significant difference between ThuLEP and HoLEP [79]. ThuLEP was associated with the shortest operative time compared with HoLEP in one of the studies [62]. Enucleated tissue weight was similar in most comparisons, except that one RCT showed that the enucleation weight was lower with GreenVEP compared with that of HoLEP.

Pang et al. in 2022 in their systematic review and meta-analysis of published RCTs comparing various techniques reported that AEEP offers similar efficacy and safety to TURP in small and medium size (30–60 grams) prostates, and it is a better alternative in large prostates when compared to open prostatectomy [47]. Improvement in IPSS, QoL, Qmax, and PVR are similar regardless of energy and technique used for the enucleation of the prostate. On comparing different EEP techniques, ThuLEP significantly improves IPSS and QoL scores more than HoLEP in the short term (1 month), but not in the longer term (12 months). There were no other functional outcome differences in meta-analyses.

Functional outcomes may well be affected by the differences in power settings, variations in the technique, and the type of morcellators used. Where laser facilities are not readily available, enucleation using plasma-kinetic energy is reported to be a good option as most of the outcomes following PKEP are like enucleation using lasers with reduced cost of the treatment.

Gauher et al. [80] in their meta-analysis reported that MoLEP performs better in terms of intraoperative outcomes when compared to traditional HoLEP. However, the difference was not clinically meaningful. It needs long-term data and multicentric trials to recommend it as a replacement for standard HoLEP. A Propensity Score-matched Analysis from the Refinement in Endoscopic Anatomical Enucleation of Prostate (REAP) Registry [81] reported that early and delayed outcomes of enucleation with ThuFLEP are comparable to those with high power HoLEP, with similar improvements in micturition parameters and IPSS. Another similar study by Kamalov AA et al. showed that ThuFLEP was comparable to bipolar enucleation in perioperative characteristics, improvement in voiding parameters, and complication rates [82].

The treatment modalities and recommendations should be tailor-made according to the prostate size, co-morbidities, and sexual needs. Before embarking on the attempts to improve the sexual outcomes of enucleation, its erectile function, ejaculatory function, and orgasmic function results need to be better defined. Exploring different ejaculatory-sparing techniques could be a golden opportunity to further consolidate the role and expand the indications of enucleation surgery. More randomized controlled trials (RCTs) are needed to compare different EEPs, and future research should focus on 'standardized' reporting, that is, reporting pre- and post-operative IPSS/IIEF and uroflowmetry parameters and using the Clavien-Dindo system for complications.

9. Conclusions

AEEP provides at least equivalent, and possibly greater improvements in urinary symptom scores, maximum urinary flow rates (Qmax), and PVR compared to vaporization and conventional resection techniques. AEEP has less bleeding and shorter catheter-free time and length of stay. AEEP is strongly recommended in large prostates because of its safety and efficacy. Overcoming the learning curve can be made easier with proper mentorship and guidance. All types of energies used for AEEP give equivalent long-term outcomes; however, HoLEP has the longest duration follow-up data and the largest published evidence in favor of successful outcomes. Newer en-bloc enucleation techniques and energy sources like TFL have promising future. AEEP is a truly well-established, size-independent gold standard, minimally invasive surgical treatment for BPH.

Conflicts of interest

The authors declare no conflict of interest.

Author details

Ajay Bhandarkar[1*], Nisarg Mehta[2] and Rishabh Handa[3]

1 Sujay Urological Hospital, Vadodara, India

2 Radiance Urology Hospital, Vadodara, India

3 Handa Urology Centre, Vadodara, India

*Address all correspondence to: adbhandarkar63@gmail.com

IntechOpen

© 2024 The Author(s). Licensee IntechOpen. This chapter is distributed under the terms of the Creative Commons Attribution License (http://creativecommons.org/licenses/by/4.0), which permits unrestricted use, distribution, and reproduction in any medium, provided the original work is properly cited. (cc) BY

References

[1] Vuichoud C, Loughlin KR. Benign prostatic hyperplasia: Epidemiology, economics, and evaluation. The Canadian Journal of Urology. 2015;**22**(Suppl. 1):1-6

[2] Coyne KS, Sexton CC, Thompson CL, et al. The prevalence of lower urinary tract symptoms (LUTS) in the USA, the UK and Sweden: Results from the epidemiology of LUTS (EpiLUTS) study. BJU International. 2009;**104**:352-360

[3] Lee DY, Kam SC. Should psychiatric symptoms Be evaluated in elderly males with lower urinary tract symptoms? International Neurourology Journal. 2023;**27**(2):155-156. DOI: 10.5213/inj.2346038.019. Epub 2023 Jun 30

[4] Gilfrich C, Leicht H, Fahlenbrach C, Jeschke E, Popken G, Stolzenburg JU, et al. Morbidity and mortality after surgery for lower urinary tract symptoms: A study of 95577 cases from a nationwide German health insurance database. Prostate Cancer and Prostatic Diseases. 2016;**19**(4):406-411. DOI: 10.1038/pcan.2016.33. Epub 2016 Aug 9

[5] Lerner LB, McVary KT, Barry MJ, Bixler BR, Dahm P, Das AK, et al. Management of Lower Urinary Tract Symptoms Attributed to benign prostatic hyperplasia: AUA GUIDELINE PART I-initial work-up and medical management. The Journal of Urology. 2021;**206**(4):806-817. DOI: 10.1097/JU.0000000000002183. Epub 2021 Aug 13. Erratum in: J Urol. 2021 Nov;206(5):1339

[6] Varkarakis I, Kyriakakis Z, Delis A, Protogerou V, Deliveliotis C. Long-term results of open transvesical prostatectomy from a contemporary series of patients. Urology. 2004;**64**:306-310

[7] Reich O, Gratzke C, Bachmann A, Seitz M, Schlenker B, Hermanek P, et al. Morbidity, mortality and early outcome of transurethral resection of the prostate: A prospective multicenter evaluation of 10,654 patients. The Journal of Urology. 2008;**180**(1):246-249. DOI: 10.1016/j.juro.2008.03.058. Epub 2008 May 21

[8] Behr A, Salleron J, Mazeaud C, Larose C, Dagry A, Balkau B, et al. Comparison of surgical procedures for benign prostatic hyperplasia of medium-volume prostates: Evaluation of the causes of rehospitalization from the French National Hospital Database (PMSI-MCO). World Journal of Urology. 2023;**41**(9):2481-2488. DOI: 10.1007/s00345-023-04509-6. Epub 2023 Aug 7

[9] Xie CY, Zhu GB, Wang XH, Liu XB. Five-year follow-up results of a randomized controlled trial comparing bipolar plasmakinetic and monopolar transurethral resection of the prostate. Yonsei Medical Journal. 2012;**53**(4):734-741. DOI: 10.3349/ymj.2012.53.4.734

[10] Fraundorfer MR, Gilling PJ. Holmium: YAG laser enucleation of the prostate combined with mechanical Morcellation: Preliminary results. European Urology. 1998;**33**(1):69-72. DOI: 10.1159/000019535

[11] Gilling PJ, Aho TF, Frampton CM, King CJ, Fraundorfer MR. Holmium laser enucleation of the prostate: Results at 6 years. European Urology. 2008;**53**(4):744-749. DOI: 10.1016/j.eururo.2007.04.052. Epub 2007 Apr 23

[12] Ibrahim A, Alharbi M, Elhilali MM, Aubé M, Carrier S. 18 years of holmium laser enucleation of the prostate: A single center experience. The Journal of Urology. 2019;**202**(4):795-800.

DOI: 10.1097/JU.0000000000000280. Epub 2019 Sep 6

[13] Neill MG, Gilling PJ, Kennett KM, Frampton CM, Westenberg AM, Fraundorfer MR, et al. Randomized trial comparing holmium laser enucleation of prostate with plasmakinetic enucleation of prostate for treatment of benign prostatic hyperplasia. Urology. 2006;**68**(5):1020-1024. DOI: 10.1016/j.urology.2006.06.021. Epub 2006 Nov 7

[14] Herrmann TRW, Gravas S, de la Rosette JJ, Wolters M, Anastasiadis AG, Giannakis I. Lasers in transurethral enucleation of the prostate-do we really need them. Journal of Clinical Medicine. 2020;**9**(5):1412. DOI: 10.3390/jcm9051412

[15] Herrmann TR. Enucleation is enucleation is enucleation is enucleation. World Journal of Urology. 2016;**34**(10):1353-1355. DOI: 10.1007/s00345-016-1922-3. Epub 2016 Sep 1

[16] Enikeev D, Misrai V, Rijo E, Sukhanov R, Chinenov D, Gazimiev M, et al. EAU, AUA and NICE guidelines on surgical and minimally invasive treatment of benign prostate hyperplasia: A critical appraisal of the guidelines using the AGREE-II tool. Urologia Internationalis. 2022;**106**(1):1-10. DOI: 10.1159/000517675

[17] Lin Y, Wu X, Xu A, et al. Transurethral enucleation of the prostate versus transvesical open prostatectomy for large benign prostatic hyperplasia: A systematic review and meta-analysis of randomized controlled trials. World Journal of Urology. 2016;**34**:1207-1219. DOI: 10.1007/s00345-015-1735-9

[18] Li M, Qiu J, Hou Q, Wang D, Huang W, Hu C, et al. Endoscopic enucleation versus open prostatectomy for treating large benign prostatic hyperplasia: A meta-analysis of randomized controlled trials. PLoS One. 2015;**10**(3):e0121265. DOI: 10.1371/journal.pone.0121265

[19] Ahyai SA, Gilling P, Kaplan SA, Kuntz RM, Madersbacher S, Montorsi F, et al. Meta-analysis of functional outcomes and complications following transurethral procedures for lower urinary tract symptoms resulting from benign prostatic enlargement. European Urology. 2010;**58**(3):384-397. DOI: 10.1016/j.eururo.2010.06.005. Epub 2010 Jun 11

[20] Zhang Y, Yuan P, Ma D, et al. Efficacy and safety of enucleation vs. resection of prostate for treatment of benign prostatic hyperplasia: A meta-analysis of randomized controlled trials. Prostate Cancer and Prostatic Diseases. 2019;**22**:493-508. DOI: 10.1038/s41391-019-0135-4

[21] Madersbacher S, Lackner J, Brössner C, Röhlich M, Stancik I, Willinger M, et al. Prostate study Group of the Austrian Society of urology. Reoperation, myocardial infarction and mortality after transurethral and open prostatectomy: A nation-wide, long-term analysis of 23,123 cases. European Urology. 2005;**47**(4):499-504. DOI: 10.1016/j.eururo.2004.12.010. Epub 2005 Jan 23

[22] Wroclawski ML, Teles SB, Amaral BS, et al. A systematic review and meta-analysis of the safety and efficacy of endoscopic enucleation and non-enucleation procedures for benign prostatic enlargement. World Journal of Urology. 2020;**38**:1663-1684. DOI: 10.1007/s00345-019-02968-4

[23] Salmivalli A, Ettala O, Boström PJ, Kytö V. Mortality after surgery for benign prostate hyperplasia: A nationwide cohort study. World Journal of Urology.

2022;**40**(7):1785-1791. DOI: 10.1007/s00345-022-03999-0. Epub 2022 Apr 16

[24] Hiraoka Y, Akimoto M. Transurethral enucleation of benign prostatic hyperplasia. The Journal of Urology. 1989;**142**(5):1247-1250. DOI: 10.1016/s0022-5347(17)39047-x

[25] Gilling PJ, Cass CB, Malcolm AR, Fraundorfer MR. Combination holmium and Nd:YAG laser ablation of the prostate: Initial clinical experience. Journal of Endourology. 1995;**9**(2):151-153. DOI: 10.1089/end.1995.9.151

[26] Hochreiter WW, Thalmann GN, Burkhard FC, Studer UE. Holmium laser enucleation of the prostate combined with electrocautery resection: The mushroom technique. The Journal of Urology. 2002;**168**(4 Pt. 1):1470-1474. DOI: 10.1016/S0022-5347(05)64476-X

[27] Liu C, Zheng S, Li H, Xu K. Transurethral enucleation and resection of prostate in patients with benign prostatic hyperplasia by plasma kinetics. The Journal of Urology. 2010;**184**(6):2440-2445. DOI: 10.1016/j.juro.2010.08.037. Epub 2010 Oct 16

[28] Hirasawa Y, Ide H, Yasumizu Y, Hoshino K, Ito Y, Masuda T. Comparison of transurethral enucletion with bipolar and transurethral resection in saline for managing benign prostatic hyperplasia. BJU International. 2012;**110**:E864-E869

[29] Geavlete B, Stanescu F, Iacoboaie C, Geavlete P. Bipolar plasma enucleation of the prostate vs open prostatectomy in large benign prostatic hyperplasia cases - A medium term, prospective, randomized comparison. BJU International. 2013;**111**(5):793-803. DOI: 10.1111/j.1464-410X.2012.11730.x. Epub 2013 Mar 7

[30] Xia S-j, Zhang Y-n, Jun L, Sun X-w, Zhang J, Zhu Y-y, et al. Thulium laser resection of prostate-tangerine technique in treatment of benign prostate hyperplasia. Zhonghua Yi Xue Za Zhi. 2005;**85**(45):3225-3228

[31] Bach T, Herrmann TR, Ganzer R, Burchardt M, Gross AJ. RevoLix vaporesection of the prostate: Initial results of 54 patients with a 1-year follow-up. World Journal of Urology. 2007;**25**(3):257-262. DOI: 10.1007/s00345-007-0171-x. Epub 2007 May 25

[32] Herrmann TRW, Bach T, Imkamp F, et al. Thulium laser enucleation of the prostate (ThuLEP): Transurethral anatomical prostatectomy with laser support. Introduction of a novel technique for the treatment of benign prostatic obstruction. World Journal of Urology. 2010;**28**:45-51. DOI: 10.1007/s00345-009-0503-0

[33] Kuntzman RS, Malek RS, Barrett DM, Bostwick DG. Potassium-titanyl-phosphate laser vaporization of the prostate: A comparative functional and pathologic study in canines. Urology. 1996;**48**(4):575-583. DOI: 10.1016/S0090-4295(96)00247-6

[34] Sancha G, Fernando VC, Rivera GG, Botsevski A, Kotsev J, Herrmann T. Common trend: Move to enucleation—Is there a case for GreenLight enucleation? Development and description of the technique. World Journal of Urology. 2015;**33**(4):539-547. DOI: 10.1007/s00345-014-1339-9

[35] Erol A, Cam K, Tekin A, et al. High power diode laservaporization of the prostate: Preliminary results forbenign prostatic hyperplasia. The Journal of Urology. 2009;**182**:1078-1082

[36] Lusuardi L, Myatt A, Sieberer M, Jeschke S, Zimmermann R, Janetschek G. Safety and efficacy of eraser laser enucleation of the prostate: Preliminary

report. The Journal of Urology. 2011;**186**(5):1967-1971. DOI: 10.1016/j.juro.2011.07.026

[37] Xu A, Zou Y, Li B, Liu C, Zheng S, Li H, et al. A randomized trial comparing diode laser enucleation of the prostate with plasmakinetic enucleation and resection of the prostate for the treatment of benign prostatic hyperplasia. Journal of Endourology. 2013;**27**(10):1254-1260. DOI: 10.1089/end.2013.0107. Epub 2013 Sep 19

[38] Zou Z, Xu A, Zheng S, Chen B, Xu Y, Li H, et al. Dual-centre randomized-controlled trial comparing transurethral endoscopic enucleation of the prostate using diode laser vs. bipolar plasmakinetic for the treatment of LUTS secondary of benign prostate obstruction: 1-year follow-up results. World Journal of Urology. 2018;**36**(7):1117-1126. DOI: 10.1007/s00345-018-2229-3. Epub 2018 Feb 19

[39] Kuntz RM, Lehrich K, Ahyai SA. Holmium laser enucleation of the prostate versus open prostatectomy for prostates greater than 100 grams: 5-year follow-up results of a randomised clinical trial. European Urology. 2008;**53**(1):160-166. DOI: 10.1016/j.eururo.2007.08.036

[40] Gilling PJ et al. Long-term results of a randomized trial comparing holmium laser enucleation of the prostate and transurethral resection of the prostate: Results at 7 years. BJU International. 2012;**109**(3):408-411. DOI: 10.1111/j.1464-410X.2011.10359.x

[41] Morozov A, Taratkin M, Shpikina A, et al. Comparison of EEP and TURP long-term outcomes: Systematic review and meta-analysis. World Journal of Urology. 2023;**41**:3471-3483. DOI: 10.1007/s00345-023-04666-8

[42] Dusing MW, Krambeck AE, Terry C, Matlaga BR, Miller NL, Humphreys MR, et al. Holmium laser enucleation of the prostate: Efficiency gained by experience and operative technique. The Journal of Urology. 2010;**184**(2):635-640. DOI: 10.1016/j.juro.2010.03.130. Epub 2010 Jun 19

[43] Oh SJ. Current surgical techniques of enucleation in holmium laser enucleation of the prostate. Investigative and Clinical Urology. 2019;**60**(5):333-342. DOI: 10.4111/icu.2019.60.5.333. Epub 2019 Aug 30

[44] Bhandarkar AM, Patel DC. Modified "en bloc" bipolar plasma enucleation of prostate: Our technique for treatment of obstructive benign prostatic hyperplasia. Videourology. 2020;**34**(2). DOI: 10.1089/vid.2019.0090 Corpus ID: 216206437

[45] Zhou J, Hua Z, Tang M, Meng X, Li P. Application of en bloc and urethral mucosal flap sparing techniques improve the functional outcomes in holmium laser enucleation of prostate: A retrospective case control study. American Journal of Men's Health. 2022;**16**(5):15579883221131412. DOI: 10.1177/15579883221131412

[46] Scoffone CM, Cracco CM. The en-bloc no-touch holmium laser enucleation of the prostate (HoLEP) technique. World Journal of Urology. 2016;**34**(8):1175-1181. DOI: 10.1007/s00345-015-1741-y

[47] Pang KH et al. Complications and functional outcomes of endoscopic enucleation of the prostate: A systematic review and meta-analysis of randomised-controlled studies. Central European Journal of Urology. 2022;**75**(4):357-386. DOI: 10.5173/ceju.2022.174

[48] Wendt-Nordahl G, Huckele S, Honeck P, et al. 980-nm diode laser: A novel laser technology for vaporization of the prostate. European Urology.

2007;**52**(6):1723-1728. DOI: 10.1016/j.eururo.2007.06.029

[49] Bhandarkar A, Patel D. Comparison of holmium laser enucleation of the prostate with bipolar Plasmakinetic enucleation of the prostate: A randomized, prospective controlled trial at midterm follow-up. Journal of Endourology. 2022;**36**(12):1567-1574. DOI: 10.1089/end.2022.0449. Epub 2022 Oct 13

[50] Taratkin M, Checcucci E, Androsov A, Azilgareeva C, Brill B, Morozov A, et al. Thulium fiber laser in BPH surgery: Bench to bedside – A systematic review on behalf of YAU urotechnology working group. Frontiers in Urology. 2022;**2**:1017069. DOI: 10.3389/fruro.2022.1017069

[51] Yilmaz M, Esser J, Kraft L, Petzold R, Sigle A, Gratzke C, et al. Experimental ex-vivo performance study comparing a novel, pulsed thulium solid-state laser, chopped thulium fibre laser, low and high-power holmium:YAG laser for endoscopic enucleation of the prostate. World Journal of Urology. 2022;**40**(2):601-606. DOI: 10.1007/s00345-021-03825-z

[52] Taratkin M, Azilgareeva C, Cacciamani GE, Enikeev D. Thulium fiber laser in urology: Physics made simple. Current Opinion in Urology. 2022;**32**(2):166-172. DOI: 10.1097/MOU.0000000000000967

[53] Moore J, Chavez A, Narang G, Bogle J, Stern K. Operating room noise hazards during laser lithotripsy: A comparison between the thulium fiber and holmium laser platforms. World Journal of Urology. 2022;**40**(3):801-805. DOI: 10.1007/s00345-021-03897-x

[54] Elhilali MM, Badaan S, Ibrahim A, Andonian S. Use of the Moses technology to improve holmium laser lithotripsy outcomes: A preclinical study. Journal of Endourology. 2017;**31**(6):598-604. DOI: 10.1089/end.2017.0050. Epub 2017 Apr 25

[55] Netsch C, Bach T, Herrmann TRW, Neubauer O, Gross AJ. Evaluation of the learning curve for thulium VapoEnucleation of the prostate (ThuVEP) using a mentor-based approach. World Journal of Urology. 2013;**31**(5):1231-1238. DOI: 10.1007/s00345-012-0894-1

[56] Enikeev D. En bloc and two-lobe techniques for laser endoscopic enucleation of the prostate: Retrospective comparative analysis of peri- and postoperative outcomes. International Urology and Nephrology. 2019;**51**(11):1969-1974. DOI: 10.1007/s1125 5-019-02259 -2

[57] Kampantais S, Dimopoulos P, Tasleem A, Acher P, Gordon K, Young A. Assessing the learning curve of holmium laser enucleation of prostate (HoLEP). A systematic review. Urology. 2018;**120**:9-22. DOI: 10.1016/j.urolo gy.2018.06.012

[58] Robert G. Multicentre prospective evaluation of the learning curve of holmium laser enucleation of the prostate (HoLEP). BJU International. 2016;**117**(3):495-499. DOI: 10.1111/bju.13124

[59] Lerner LB, Tyson MD, Mendoza PJ. Stress incontinence during the learning curve of holmium laser enucleation of the prostate. Journal of Endourology. 2010;**24**(10):1655-1658. DOI: 10.1089/end.2010.0021

[60] Peyronnet B. Learning curves and perioperative outcomes after endoscopic enucleation of the prostate: A comparison between GreenLight 532-nm and holmium lasers. World Journal of Urology. 2017;**35**(6):973-983. DOI: 10.1007/s0034 5-016-1957-5

[61] Saredi G. Evaluation of the learning curve for thulium laser enucleation of the prostate with the aid of a simulator tool but without tutoring: Comparison of two surgeons with different levels of endoscopic experience endourology and technology. BMC Urology. 2015;**15**(1):7. DOI: 10.1186/s1289 4-015-0045-2

[62] Enikeev D. A randomized trial comparing the learning curve of 3 endoscopic enucleation techniques (HoLEP, ThuFLEP, and MEP) for BPH using mentoring approach—Initial results. Urology. 2018;**121**:51-57. DOI: 10.1016/j.urolo gy.2018.06.045

[63] Enikeev D, Morozov A, Taratkin M, Misrai V, Rijo E, Podoinitsin A, et al. Systematic review of the endoscopic enucleation of the prostate learning curve. World Journal of Urology. 2021;**39**(7):2427-2438. DOI: 10.1007/s00345-020-03451-1. Epub 2020 Sep 17

[64] Xiong W, Sun M, Ran Q, Chen F, Du Y, Dou K. Learning curve for bipolar transurethral enucleation and resection of the prostate in saline for symptomatic benign prostatic hyperplasia: Experience in the first 100 consecutive patients. Urologia Internationalis. 2013;**90**(1):68-74. DOI: 10.1159/000343235

[65] Shigemura K, Tanaka K, Yamamichi F, Chiba K, Fujisawa M. Comparison of predictive factors for postoperative incontinence of holmium laser enucleation of the prostate by the surgeons' experience during learning curve. International Neurourology Journal. 2016;**20**(1):59-68. DOI: 10.5213/inj.1630396.198

[66] Cornwell LB, Smith GE, Paonessa JE. Predictors of postoperative urinary incontinence after holmium laser enucleation of the prostate: 12 months follow-up. Urology. 2019;**124**:213-217. DOI: 10.1016/j.urology.2018.11.032. Epub 2018 Dec 4

[67] Krambeck AE, Handa SE, Lingeman JE. Experience with more than 1,000 holmium laser prostate enucleations for benign prostatic hyperplasia. The Journal of Urology. 2010;**183**:1105

[68] Xu N, Chen S-H, Xue X-Y, Wei Y, Zheng Q-S, Li X-D, et al. Older age and larger prostate volume are associated with stress urinary incontinence after plasmakinetic enucleation of the prostate. BioMed Research International. 2017;**2017**:1-6, 6923290. DOI: 10.1155/2017/6923290

[69] Elmansy HM, Kotb A, Elhilali MM. Holmium laser enucleation of the prostate: Long-term durability of clinical outcomes and complication rates during 10 years of followup. The Journal of Urology. 2011;**186**(5):1972-1976. DOI: 10.1016/j.juro.2011.06.065. Epub 2011 Sep 23

[70] Placer J, Gelabert-Mas A, Vallmanya F, Manresa JM, Menéndez V, Cortadellas R, et al. Holmium laser enucleation of prostate: Outcome and complications of self-taught learning curve. Urology. 2009;**73**(5):1042-1048. DOI: 10.1016/j.urology.2008.12.052. ISSN 0090-4295

[71] Romero-Otero J, Garcia-Gonzalez L, Garcia-Gomez B, Justo-Quintas J, Garcia-Rojo E, Gonzalez-Padilla DA, et al. Factors influencing intraoperative blood loss in patients undergoing holmium laser enucleation of the prostate (HoLEP) for benign prostatic hyperplasia: A large multicenter analysis. Urology. 2019;**132**:177-182. DOI: 10.1016/j.urology.2019.06.024

[72] Naspro R, Suardi N, Salonia A, Scattoni V, Guazzoni G, Colombo R, et al. Holmium laser enucleation of the

prostate versus open prostatectomy for prostates >70 g: 24-month follow-up. European Urology. 2006;**50**(3):563-568. DOI: 10.1016/j.eururo.2006.04.003

[73] Shah HN, Mahajan AP, Hegde SS, Bansal MB. Peri-operative complications of holmium laser enucleation of the prostate: Experience in the first 280 patients, and a review of literature. BJU International. 2007;**100**(1):94-101. DOI: 10.1111/j.1464-410X.2007.06867.x

[74] Montorsi F, Naspro R, Salonia A, Suardi N, Briganti A, Zanoni M, et al. Holmium laser enucleation versus transurethral resection of the prostate: Results from a 2-Center prospective randomized trial in patients with obstructive benign prostatic hyperplasia. The Journal of Urology. 2008;**179** (Suppl. 5):S87-S90. DOI: 10.1016/j.juro.2008.03.143

[75] Zhang J, Zhenyu O, Zhang X, He W, Wang R, Mo M, et al. Holmium laser enucleation of the prostate versus thulium laser enucleation of the prostate for the treatment of large-volume prostates > 80 ml: 18-month follow-up results. World Journal of Urology. 2020;**38**(6):1555-1562. DOI: 10.1007/s00345-019-02945-x

[76] Gravas S, Gacci M, Gratzke C, Herrmann TRW, Karavitakis M, Kyriazis I, et al. Summary paper on the 2023 European association of urology guidelines on the Management of non-neurogenic male lower urinary tract symptoms. European Urology. 2023;**84**(2):207-222. DOI: 10.1016/j.eururo.2023.04.008. Epub 2023 May 17

[77] Ma Y, Lin L, Luo Z, Jin T. Network meta-analysis of the treatment safety and efficacy of different lasers in prostate enucleation. Journal of Endourology. 2022;**36**(12):1613-1624. DOI: 10.1089/end.2022.0282. Epub 2022 Sep 26

[78] Zhang F, Shao Q, Herrmann TR, et al. Thulium laser versus holmium laser transurethral enucleation of the prostate: 18-month follow-up data of a single center. Urology. 2012;**79**(4):869-874. DOI: 10.1016/j.urology.2011.12.018

[79] Hartung FO, Kowalewski KF, von Hardenberg J, Worst TS, Kriegmair MC, Nuhn P, et al. Holmium versus thulium laser enucleation of the prostate: A systematic review and meta-analysis of randomized controlled trials. European Urology Focus. 2022;**8**(2):545-554. DOI: 10.1016/j.euf.2021.03.024. Epub 2021 Apr 8

[80] Gauhar V, Gilling P, Pirola GM, Chan VW, Lim EJ, Maggi M, et al. Does MOSES technology enhance the efficiency and outcomes of standard holmium laser enucleation of the prostate? Results of a systematic review and meta-analysis of comparative studies. European Urology Focus. 2022;**8**(5):1362-1369. DOI: 10.1016/j.euf.2022.01.013. Epub 2022 Jan 31

[81] Gauhar V, Nedbal C, Castellani D, Fong KY, Sofer M, Socarrás MR, et al. Comparison between thulium fiber laser and high-power holmium laser for anatomic endoscopic enucleation of the prostate: A propensity score-matched analysis from the REAP registry. European Urology Focus. 2024;**10**(1):182-188. DOI: 10.1016/j.euf.2023.06.009. Epub 2023 Jul 4

[82] Kamalov AA, Sorokin NI, Dzitiev VK, Strigunov AA, Nesterova OY, Bondar IV. Propensity score-matched analysis comparing perioperative, functional, and safety outcomes between thulium fiber laser and bipolar enucleation of the prostate performed by a single surgeon with two years of follow-up. Investigative and Clinical Urology. 2024;**65**(2):139-147. DOI: 10.4111/icu.20230270

Chapter 4

Challenging the Gold Standard Transurethral Resection of the Prostate with Holmium Laser Enucleation in the Treatment of Benign Prostatic Hyperplasia: Paradigm Shift in Northern Cyprus

Necmi Bayraktar

Abstract

Benign prostatic hyperplasia (BPH) is a common condition among men over the age of 50, which can significantly impact their quality of life. Transurethral Resection of the Prostate (TURP) has long been considered the gold standard for the surgical treatment of BPH because of its effectiveness and integration into urology training. However, in recent years, Holmium Laser Enucleation of the Prostate (HoLEP) has gained popularity owing to reduced bleeding, shorter hospitalization, and faster recovery times. This study aimed to evaluate the transition from TURP to HoLEP among urologists at Burhan Nalbantoğlu State Hospital by analyzing learning curves, complication rates, and patient outcomes. The study results suggest that HoLEP offers several advantages over TURP, including shorter hospital stay and lower postoperative complications, although it requires significant training and investment. Overall, this study supports HoLEP as a promising alternative to TURP, reflecting a shift in the paradigm of BPH management.

Keywords: benign prostatic hyperplasia (BPH), transurethral resection of the prostate (TURP), holmium laser enucleation (HoLEP), laser prostatectomy, urology, minimally invasive surgery, learning curve, postoperative complications, patient outcomes

1. Introduction

Benign prostatic hyperplasia (BPH) is a prevalent condition among the elderly male population that can cause lower urinary tract symptoms (LUTS) by impeding urine flow. This can have a substantial influence on the patients' quality of life. Epidemiological studies have shown that approximately 50% of men in their 50s and up to 90% of men in their 80s are affected by BPH [1]. In the past, traditional surgical procedures such as Transurethral Resection of the Prostate (TURP) and open prostatectomy for significant prostates have been favored for BPH treatment. However, advancements in surgical techniques and technological progress have led to the emergence of less-invasive methods, the most noteworthy of which is Holmium Laser Enucleation (HoLEP) [2, 3].

For several years, the Transurethral Resection of the Prostate (TURP) has been widely regarded as the gold standard treatment for Benign Prostatic Hyperplasia (BPH). TURP was first introduced in the early twentieth century and has since made significant advances. Initially, the removal of prostate tissue using a resectoscope was refined over the years with improvements in devices and techniques [4]. This procedure, which involves the removal of prostate tissue using a resectoscope inserted through the urethra, has undergone significant advancements since its inception in the early twentieth century. Several factors have contributed to TURP being considered the gold standard. Efficacy is one reason for this. Rapid regression of symptoms and improvement in patients' quality of life following prostate tissue removal are among the benefits of this procedure. The widespread acceptance of TURP is due to the experience gained over many years, which has increased the confidence in the method. The experience and reliability of the method have contributed to its success. Numerous studies have documented the long-term effectiveness of TURP [5–7]. Transurethral Resection of the Prostate (TURP) is widely regarded as a fundamental aspect of urological education, and as such, it is both accessible and widely available. Moreover, when considering the investment required for equipment and devices, TURP is a more cost-effective option than other more recent methods (**Table 1**).

Transurethral Resection of the Prostate (TURP) is a minimally invasive surgical procedure rooted in urologists' efforts to minimize surgical invasiveness. In 2018, a study by MJ Young et al. examined the advancements in TURP techniques and traced the historical development of this treatment approach from its origins to the present day [4]. Transurethral Resection of the Prostate (TURP) has exhibited substantial advancements in both safety and efficacy; however, the procedure still presents certain challenges and intricacies. Although Transurethral Resection of the Prostate (TURP) has been established as a safe and effective therapy for Benign Prostatic Hyperplasia (BPH), a proficient surgeon must prevent potential complications and

Reason	Explanation
Efficiency	Transurethral Resection of the Prostate (TURP) is a highly effective procedure that removes prostate tissue to enhance urine flow and alleviate symptoms, such as difficulty urinating.
Experience and reliability	It has decades of clinical use with a proven track record, giving doctors confidence.
Long-term outcomes	Long-term relief from symptoms associated with benign prostatic hyperplasia (BPH) has been demonstrated to be durably provided by transurethral resection of the prostate (TURP), as per findings from studies.
Standardized training	TURP is a crucial component of urological training and is widely performed and accessible.
Cost effectiveness	TURP is often the more economical choice in various areas because of lower equipment costs compared to other treatments.

Table 1.
Reasons for considering TURP as the gold standard in BPH treatment.

attain optimal results. Transurethral Resection of the Prostate (TURP) has gained considerable popularity in the mid-twentieth century as a treatment for benign prostatic hyperplasia (BPH). Technological advancements, including the development of modern instruments such as the Stern-McCarthy resectoscope in the 1930s, which improved optics and irrigation systems to enable better visualization and operational capabilities within the prostate, have contributed to the enhanced effectiveness of TURP [8]. A study conducted by CE Hawtrey and RD Williams in 2008 provided a comprehensive account of the evolution of TURP at the University of Iowa. This study documented the historical development of the procedure and its applications throughout various time periods, which facilitated a deeper understanding of TURP's role of TURP in the field of surgical urology [9].

Holmium Laser Enucleation of the Prostate (HoLEP) was initially performed by Dr. Peter Gilling in New Zealand in 1997. This procedure is a minimally invasive technique that aims to alleviate bladder obstruction by removing the inner prostate tissue. HoLEP has emerged as an effective treatment option, particularly for large prostates, and offers several advantages over conventional methods such as transurethral resection of the prostate (TURP) [10].

In 1999, Dr. James Lingeman introduced Holmium Laser Enucleation of the Prostate (HoLEP) to the United States, which has since become the gold standard treatment for benign prostatic hyperplasia (BPH). HoLEP is recognized as the only surgical intervention that can be performed regardless of the size of the prostate. This characteristic of HoLEP makes it a highly appealing option for patients with larger prostates, who may not be suitable candidates for other surgical procedures.

Recently, the emergence of alternative treatment options, particularly laser therapy and medications, has called into question the traditional role of TURP in BPH management. Nevertheless, TURP continues to be a widely performed surgical procedure and has been continually refined through advancements in surgical techniques and equipment. Despite the development of minimally invasive procedures, TURP remains a popular surgical intervention because of its well-established effectiveness and versatility in the treatment of various urological conditions.

The history of Transurethral Resection of the Prostate (TURP) embodies the continuous evolution of medicine and the pursuit of more effective, safer, and minimally invasive treatments for benign prostatic hyperplasia (BPH). This journey exemplifies the progress made in medical technology and transformation of patient care. Nevertheless, it is crucial to acknowledge that these technological advancements have engendered new impediments pertaining to healthcare accessibility and affordability for numerous individuals.

1.1 The situation in the TRNC and the change of methodology

In the TRNC, there has been an important paradigm shift in the treatment of BPH, especially in health institutions, such as Burhan Nalbantoğlu State Hospital. The transition from traditional TURP and open prostatectomy to HoLEP surgery has led to significant improvements in both hospital practices and patient outcomes. These advancements have reduced perioperative complications, shortened recovery times, and improved patient satisfaction. Additionally, HoLEP allows for a more precise and minimally invasive approach, further enhancing the benefits of this procedure over traditional methods. Implementing this modification has resulted in a decrease in the duration of hospital stay, a decline in the incidence of complications, and an increase in patient satisfaction and confidence levels in surgical procedures [2].

1.2 Literature review and current developments

According to a research conducted by Elmansy et al. in 2023, HoLEP has become widely recognized as a minimally invasive surgical option for the management of BPH. This study demonstrated that HoLEP is effective for prostate sizes ranging from small to large and offers several advantages over TURP, including a reduced risk of bleeding and a more rapid recovery time [2]. Furthermore, HoLEP is a minimally invasive procedure that utilizes a high-energy holmium laser to remove the prostate tissue, which results in precise and effective removal of the obstructive tissue, thereby improving the patient's urinary symptoms. Additionally, HoLEP has been shown to be effective in treating patients with benign prostatic hyperplasia (BPH) and can be performed on an outpatient basis, making it a convenient option for many patients. Overall, the benefits of HoLEP make it a promising alternative to TURP and other traditional surgical procedures for BPH treatment. According to a study conducted by Elkoushy et al. in 2015, the necessity for reoperation following HoLEP is minimal and the long-term safety and efficacy of this method are evident [3]. Elkoushy et al. [3] emphasized the potential of HoLEP as a viable alternative to traditional surgical methods for the treatment of benign prostatic hyperplasia (BPH). This is attributed to its high success rate, low rate of complications, and minimal need for long-term reintervention. These findings have significant ramifications for the management of BPH and could potentially enhance the quality of life of patients with this condition.

1.3 Economic assessment

Although the HoLEP procedure has high initial costs, it improves the overall efficiency of patient care and saves costs for the healthcare system in the long run. Shorter hospital stays and lower complication rates allow for a more efficient use of hospital resources [2]. For instance, several studies found that patients who underwent a same-day surgery protocol had shorter hospital stays and lower complication rates than those who underwent traditional hospitalization procedures, demonstrating the potential benefits of more efficient use of hospital resources [11, 12].

The objective of this research was to thoroughly investigate the transition from traditional TURP to HoLEP in the management of BPH and to emphasize the progress, challenges, and consequences of this significant shift in paradigm. This chapter aims to deliver a comprehensive summary of the altering treatment landscape for BPH in North Cyprus by examining the clinical results and patient feedback linked to HoLEP, underlining the necessity of persistent innovation and education in urological practice.

2. Methodology

In the process of transitioning from traditional transurethral resection of the prostate (TURP) to holmium laser enucleation of the prostate (HoLEP), this study evaluated the conversion of experienced urologists. The learning curves and performance improvements of seven physicians who had access to the holmium laser device at Burhan Nalbantoğlu State Hospital were analyzed, as well as the patient series and treatment outcomes of seven physicians who began performing HoLEP at the hospital in 2022. The aforementioned urologists, A, B, C, D, E, F, and G, possess comparable qualifications in general urology, with each having a distinct focus on endourology based on their varying years of urology residency experience. Specifically, A has 16 years, B has 17 years, C has 27 years, D has 9 years, E has 2 years, F has 15 years, and G has 24 years of experience. A total of 216 surgical cases for benign prostatic hyperplasia (BPH) were included in the study. Information regarding physicians' procedure preferences, order of procedures, procedure duration, complications, and recovery time was recorded. Time-series analysis was employed to evaluate changes in procedure duration, complication rates, and recovery times for physicians from the first to the last procedure. Similarly, learning curves are drawn to illustrate how physicians' performance improves as their experience with the procedures increases. Changes in patients' surgical preference requests following 6 months of adaptation and the first holmium laser enucleation of the prostate (HoLEP) cases will also be reflected in the paradigm results.

3. Exclusion criteria

Physicians who perform HoLEP are free to employ any technique they deem appropriate, regardless of whether it involves two-lobe or en bloc resection, regardless of the size of the prostate. Physicians are not bound by any specific guidelines or criteria when selecting patients for the HoLEP. The decision to perform HoLEP was entirely left up to the physician's discretion and personal preferences. Two of the physicians had prior experience with HoLEP before 2022, but this was not considered an exclusion criterion during the transition from TURP to HoLEP. The patient can request a procedure for benign prostate enlargement; however, the final decision is made by the urologist responsible for the patient. Patients with neurogenic bladder and/or suspected neurogenic bladder were excluded from the study.

3.1 Surgical technique details

Patients were required to provide informed consent prior to surgery. During the procedure, a 26 F resectoscope sheath was used for both HoLEP and TURP procedures. HoLEP was performed through a combination of 2 and/or 3 lobe prostatectomy and en bloc, with the specific approach chosen based on factors such as the surgeon's level of experience, prostate size, and education level. Initiating a procedure with an early apical release is a key consideration. Furthermore, it was not prohibited for certain urologists to conduct blunt dissection, while others chose to perform no-touch dissection or a combination of both. For TURP cases, monopolar energy was used for instances where the prostate size was 90 g or less.

3.2 Patient preferences and demands

Prior to the initiation of Holmium Laser Enucleation of the Prostate (HoLEP) surgery at the State Hospital, the first HoLEP procedure in the Turkish Republic of Northern Cyprus (TRNC) was performed at a private medical facility, leading to the formation of a patient group with extensive knowledge and surgical experience. Consequently, it was hypothesized that changes in patient preferences and demand for surgical options could be assessed by conducting HoLEP surgery at a public hospital. An analysis of modifications in patient preferences for surgical options during the six-month adjustment period following the initial HoLEP procedure was conducted to determine the acceptance of HoLEP and its impact on patient outcomes.

4. Analysis methods

4.1 Time series analysis and learning curves

Temporal changes in procedure duration, complication rates, and recovery times from the initial to the final procedure for each urologist were assessed using time series analysis. This analysis provides insights into the evolution of urologists' performance over time. Learning curves were constructed to demonstrate the improvement in physician performance as the volume of procedures increased. These curves visually represent the improvement in procedure time and outcomes that can be achieved as physicians gain experience. The primary outcomes were the duration of surgery, intraoperative and postoperative complications, length of hospital stay, and patient recovery times. The secondary outcomes included patient satisfaction and reoperation rates. Statistical comparisons between the TURP and HoLEP groups were performed using independent t-tests for continuous variables and chi-squared tests for categorical variables.

5. Results

Between September 2022 and February 2024, 216 surgical interventions were performed for benign prostatic hyperplasia. The mean age of the patients who participated in the study was 69.4 ± 16.2 years. The allocation of patients seeking surgical or nonsurgical intervention at the time of admission was 64% HoLEP, 22% physician's discretion, and 14% treatment with medication or alternative medicine. Specifically, 67 (31%) patients underwent transurethral resection of the prostate, 139 (64.3%) underwent holmium laser enucleation of the prostate, 7 (3.24%) underwent open prostatectomy, and 3 (1.38%) underwent laparoscopic urethra-sparing prostatectomy. Urologists were found to lack adequate experience in HoLEP and Laparoscopic urethro-sparing procedures. On the other hand, all physicians were proficient and skilled in performing open prostatectomy and TURP. Of the seven urologists who performed active prostate surgeries, only five performed the HoLEP procedure. The distribution of surgeries conducted according to urologist codes is shown in **Table 2**.

	Urologist codes							
	A	**B**	**C**	**D**	**E**	**F**	**G**	**Total**
TURP*	2	4	28	16	3	3	11	67
HoLEP**	47	31	22	23	16	0	0	139
Open***	0	0	4	2	0	0	1	7
Laparoscopic****	3	0	0	0	0	0	0	3
Total	52	35	54	41	19	3	12	216

**Transuretral resection of the prostate.*
***Holmium laser enucleation of prostate.*
****Open prostatectomy.*
*****Laparoscopic urethral sparing prostatectomy.*

Table 2.
Distribution of surgeries conducted according to urologist codes.

Based on the initial procedures of the five physicians (A, B, C, D, and E) who performed the Holep procedures, it was observed that operative times gradually decreased in a sequential manner. There was a positive correlation between the training curve and time series analysis. As shown in **Figure 1**, each physician's operative time changed as they gained experience with the Holep procedure. The curve, constructed using a linear regression model, represents the overall reduction in operating times for each physician. According to the equation on the curve, the duration of surgery decreased as the order of the procedure increased. An R^2 value of 0.311 accounted for 31.1% of the model's data points.

The graph shows the operation times of the five physicians (A, B, C, D, and E) who started to perform the HoLEP procedure in Burhan Nalbantoğlu State Hospital in 2022, in the order of procedure. A linear regression model was used to determine the overall decreasing trend in the operation times of each physician (R^2 = 0.311), and the duration of hospitalization and catheterization times were evaluated for TURP and HoLEP procedures. The mean length of stay was 3.49 ± 0.84 days for TURP and 2.41 ± 1.17 days for HoLEP. The results of the independent T test indicated a significant difference between the two procedures ($p < 0.01$). This suggests that, on average, patients stayed in the hospital for approximately 1.075 days less time after HoLEP procedures than after TURP procedures (95% confidence interval of the difference: 0.79292 to 1.35762 days). Cohen's d effect size was 1.07 (95% confidence interval of the difference lower 0.690, upper 1.305).

No instances of permanent incontinence were documented in any patient or procedure. Transient stress incontinence occurred in 28% of HoLEP cases during the 3-week to 17-week postoperative period, 16.4% of TURP patients during the 1–3-week period, 42% of open prostatectomy patients during the 1–5-week period, and no cases were reported in laparoscopic urethra-sparing prostatectomy patients. In 14.9% of the TURP cases, postoperative bleeding necessitated extended irrigation and continuous

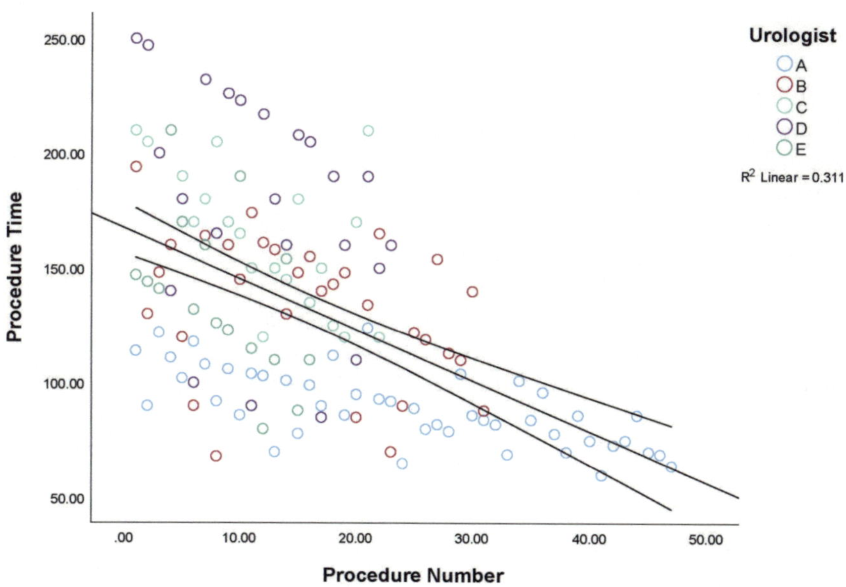

Figure 1.
Learning curves of urologists in the Transition from Transurethral Resection (TURP) to Holmium Laser Enucleation (HoLEP).

	Transurethral procedures	
Complications	**TURP (%)**	**HoLEP (%)**
Transient incontinence	16.4	28
Bleeding	14.9	4.3
TUR syndrome	NIL	NIL
Postoperative fever	NIL	12.2
Injury of prostate capsule	11.9	59.7
Conversion to open surgery	NIL	1.4

Table 3.
A summary of general complications for transurethral procedures.

monitoring. Among these patients, 30% were readmitted to the operating room, and bleeding control was established. Postoperative bleeding was identified in 4.31% (six patients) of the HoLEP cases, and only one (16.6%) of these patients received bleeding control during surgery. Only two patients in the TURP group required blood transfusions. No TUR syndrome requiring additional treatment or prolonged hospitalization was observed in any of the patients. Postoperative fever was observed in 12.2% (17 patients) in the HoLEP group. No postoperative fever was observed in the TURP group. During the procedure, 11.9% of patients who underwent transurethral resection of the prostate (TURP) experienced prostatic capsule injury, affecting a total of eight individuals. In contrast, 59.7% of patients who underwent holmium laser enucleation of the prostate (HoLEP) experienced this complication. In the HoLEP group, two patients required open surgery because of injury. A summary of general complications is presented in **Table 3**.

6. Discussion

Benign prostatic hyperplasia (BPH) is a prevalent condition among men, particularly those over the age of 50 years, and can adversely affect their quality of life. Although it is typically not a life-threatening condition, it can result in various complications if left untreated. In addition to medical therapies, surgical treatment options are also available for BPH. Among these surgical methods, Transurethral Resection of the Prostate (TURP) is widely regarded as the gold standard and an essential component of urology training programs. Consequently, most urologists acquired proficiency in TURP as part of their professional development. However, in the past decade, there has been a noticeable shift toward minimally invasive laser prostatectomy techniques, such as Holmium Laser Enucleation (HoLEP), which utilizes high-energy lasers [13]. Laser prostatectomies offer several benefits, including reduced bleeding, shorter duration of catheter and hospital stay, accelerated recovery, and early socialization [14]. Although these methods have certain advantages, they also have drawbacks. For instance, the training process can be quite challenging and expensive to undertake [15].

In terms of surgical techniques, TURP and HoLEP differ in their underlying principles. TURP begins at the bladder neck, extends to the apical lobes, and preserves the sphincter by removing parts of the prostatic urethra and capsule. In contrast, HoLEP and other laser prostatectomies preserve the apical sphincter and approach the bladder neck directly, creating a plan between the prostatic capsule and prostate adenoma [16]. From a urological perspective, the HoLEP procedure is regarded as a reverse approach for specialists who are experienced and skilled in performing TURP. According to our perspective, the primary challenge for novices arises from this detrimental approach. Additionally, initiating this procedure in clinics where there is insufficient utilization of a skilled urologist proficient in HoLEP presents another difficulty.

Research indicates that HoLEP has several benefits over TURP. In addition, according to Shvero et al. [13], HoLEP is the contemporary gold standard for surgical management of BPH and has an impressive efficacy and safety profile. Additionally, Frieben et al. [16] found that laser procedures, such as HoLEP, reduced postoperative sexual dysfunction compared with TURP.

Furthermore, Lokeshwar et al. [14] reported that laser-based treatments, including HoLEP, are preferred owing to their minimally invasive nature and low complication rates. Malaeb et al., examining surgical trends in the United States, reported an increased acceptance of laser treatments compared to TURP [17]. Similarly, Patel and Bariol examined BPH surgical treatment trends in Australia and showed that the shift to laser procedures reflects their increasing acceptance in clinical practice [15].

Our research focused on a limited time frame, thus precluding any meaningful assessment of the necessity for re-intervention. Nevertheless, it is widely accepted that HoLEP demonstrates a lower incidence of reoperation than TURP. Several investigations have indicated that the reoperation rate for HoLEP is less than 1%, while the rate for TURP is approximately 7.4% [18, 19]. HoLEP has been shown to be superior owing to its more comprehensive removal of prostate tissue, resulting in more effective relief of BPH symptoms. Additionally, HoLEP presents fewer risks of bleeding and shorter catheterization times as compared to other procedures. A consistent finding among studies is that HoLEP has lower long-term reoperation rates than TURP. Consequently, HoLEP is considered a preferable option, particularly in patients with larger prostates.

We assessed the learning curve in our study, which is common in many other studies, by evaluating the difficulty level. Experienced physicians who have undergone Transurethral Resection of the Prostate (TURP) for many years may be able to perform conscious and controlled enucleation in a certain number of patients. Moreover, 64% of patients who underwent surgery for benign prostatic hyperplasia (BPH) switched to holmium laser enucleation of the prostate (HoLEP), indicating a high level of confidence in the technique and a willingness to learn it. Notably, the number of urologists in our department who had no prior experience with laser prostatectomy and have since switched to this new method has been increasing over time. The low R2 in the time series analysis seems to be related to the size of the prostate, technical problems during surgery, other patient-related factors, and the skill of the urologists and their ability to improve this skill. Research on the assessment of the learning curve for Holmium Laser Enucleation of the Prostate (HoLEP) and Transurethral Resection (TURP) procedures is similar to our study. Although HoLEP has a long learning curve, it has been embraced by skilled surgeons. For instance, Dogan and Yildiz indicated that HoLEP was more effective in treating larger prostate glands and is regarded as an alternative to TURP by experienced practitioners [18]. In a study conducted by Eaton et al., the authors compared the learning curve between HoLEP and TURP procedures and highlighted that HoLEP demonstrates a lower complication rate despite facing technical challenges [19]. According to Shigemura et al., the learning curve of HoLEP demonstrates substantial progress in surgeons' performance as experience accumulates, and it exhibits lower complication rates compared to TURP [20].

Over the past few years, our department has performed 70–100 prostate surgeries annually. However, since we began offering the HoLEP procedure, we have observed a substantial increase in demand by 64% and a corresponding decrease in the need for reoperation. Consequently, physicians are more likely to perform laser prostatectomy. In fact, we estimate that the number of patients undergoing surgery in public hospitals has risen by 30–45% annually. These findings suggest that HoLEP enhances both efficacy and patient satisfaction in the treatment of benign prostatic hyperplasia (BPH). According to Bright and Abrams' study, HoLEP resulted in high patient satisfaction and low re-surgery rates [21].

One of the factors contributing to this increase is that HoLEP presents fewer complications and better long-term outcomes than TURP. Furthermore, although HoLEP has a steep learning curve, it is rapidly embraced by seasoned surgeons, and successful results are achieved, which amplifies its appeal. Although the learning curve for HoLEP is lengthy, its adoption by skilled surgeons in a timely manner and the attainment of positive results increase its demand. According to Shigemura et al., the learning curve for HoLEP significantly improves with greater experience and boasts lower complication rates than TURP [20]. Although this study employed a cross-sectional design, it is important to recognize its limitations. Future research incorporating additional data and more refined methods may yield a more comprehensive understanding of these issues.

HoLEP stands out compared to other surgical techniques for benign prostatic hyperplasia (BPH) owing to its reduced complication rates and faster recovery times. In our study, prostate capsule injury was more commonly reported among patients who underwent HoLEP than among those who underwent Transurethral Resection of the Prostate (TURP). However, the higher rate can be attributed to the surgeon's level of experience. While the average time for urethral catheterization was slightly shorter for HoLEP patients, many studies have reported catheter-free discharge within 24 h after the procedure. The differences in perioperative capsule injury and catheterization time are expected to decrease as the number of cases and surgeon experience increases. In addition, Elkoushy et al., HoLEP resulted in significantly lower complication rates and faster recovery times than other surgical options [3]. Patients who underwent HoLEP could resume their social lives more quickly, and bleeding complications were significantly reduced. Another study by Gilling et al., reported that HoLEP provided a lower bleeding risk and shorter catheterization time than TURP [22]. These findings suggest that HoLEP is a safer and more effective BPH treatment option and that complication rates will continue to decrease as more experienced surgeons perform the procedure.

Holmium Laser Enucleation of the Prostate (HoLEP) surgery may have higher initial costs than Transurethral Resection of the Prostate (TURP), but its long-term benefits can be economically favorable due to the absence of residual tissue, early discharge, and rapid recovery. HoLEP is also effective in treating larger prostates, while traditional methods like open prostatectomy may require longer hospital stays and result in additional expenses, such as constant incontinence and erectile dysfunction. HoLEP does not impair sexual function, does not lead to permanent incontinence, and necessitates a shorter hospital stay, making it a superior option with numerous advantages. However, our study, with a short-term focus, is insufficient to report long-term outcomes. A cost-effective analysis conducted by Erman et al. found HoLEP to be economically advantageous in the long term due to fewer complications and a lower need for re-intervention [23]. Similarly, Lokeshwar et al. reported that HoLEP preserved sexual function and had lower complication rates compared to TURP [14]. HoLEP has been found to be especially effective in large prostates, with shorter hospitalization times and lower complication rates compared to conventional methods, increasing patient satisfaction, as reported by Gilling et al. [22]. From an economic point of view, although initial costs are high, HoLEP requires fewer reoperations and patients are discharged faster, saving the healthcare system costs in the long run [24]. Furthermore, HoLEP's more complete removal of prostate tissue more effectively relieves benign prostatic hyperplasia (BPH) symptoms and contributes to lower long-term reoperation rates [20]. The long-term benefits of HoLEP offset the initial costs, making it a more economical option for the health system.

7. Conclusion

This research highlights a noteworthy change from Transurethral Resection of the Prostate (TURP) to Holmium Laser Enucleation of the Prostate (HoLEP) in the treatment of Benign Prostatic Hyperplasia (BPH) at Burhan Nalbantoğlu State Hospital in Northern Cyprus. Our results demonstrate that HoLEP offers various benefits over TURP, including shorter stays in the hospital, diminished postoperative complications, and more rapid recovery times. Although HoLEP involves a steep learning curve and extensive training, it is increasingly being recognized as the new gold standard in BPH treatment. Its superior patient outcomes and heightened satisfaction levels suggest its potential to replace TURP as the preferred surgical approach for BPH management. The shift to HoLEP represents a significant development in urological surgery, offering patients an improved quality of life.

Author details

Necmi Bayraktar
Burhan Nalbantoglu State Hospital, Nicosia, TRNC

*Address all correspondence to: necmibayraktar@icloud.com

IntechOpen

© 2024 The Author(s). Licensee IntechOpen. This chapter is distributed under the terms of the Creative Commons Attribution License (http://creativecommons.org/licenses/by/4.0), which permits unrestricted use, distribution, and reproduction in any medium, provided the original work is properly cited.

References

[1] Berry SJ et al. The development of human benign prostatic hyperplasia with age. The Journal of Urology. 1984;**132**(3):474-479

[2] Elmansy H et al. Top-down holmium laser enucleation of the prostate (HoLEP) versus traditional HoLEP for the treatment of benign prostatic hyperplasia (BPH): 1-year outcomes of a randomized controlled trial. Prostate Cancer and Prostatic Diseases. 2023:1-7. DOI: 10.1038/s41391-023-00730-x

[3] Elkoushy MA, Elshal AM, Elhilali MM. Reoperation after holmium laser Enucleation of the prostate for Management of Benign Prostatic Hyperplasia: Assessment of risk factors with time to event analysis. Journal of Endourology. 2015;**29**(7):797-804

[4] Young M et al. The changing practice of transurethral resection of the prostate. The Annals of the Royal College of Surgeons of England. 2018;**100**(4):326-329

[5] Taylor BL, Jaffe WI. Electrosurgical transurethral resection of the prostate and transurethral incision of the prostate (monopolar techniques). The Canadian Journal of Urology. 2015;**22**(Suppl. 1):24-29

[6] Prasetyo ZA, Budaya TN, Daryanto B. Characteristics of benign prostatic hyperplasia (BPH) patients undergoing transurethral resection of the prostate (TURP). Jurnal Kedokteran Brawijaya. 2021;**31**(4):220-223

[7] Rühle A, Blarer J, Oehme F, Marini L, Mattei A, Stucki P, et al. Safety and effectiveness of bipolar transurethral resection of the prostate in patients under Ongoing Oral anticoagulation with Coumarins or antiplatelet drug therapy compared to patients without anticoagulation/antiplatelet therapy. Journal of Endourology. 2019;**33**(6):455-462

[8] Marszalek M et al. Transurethral resection of the prostate. European Urology Supplements. 2009;**8**(6):504-512

[9] Hawtrey CE, Williams RD. Historical evolution of transurethral resection at the University of Iowa: Alcock and flocks. The Journal of Urology. 2008;**180**(1):55-61

[10] Gilling PJ et al. Holmium laser enucleation of the prostate (HoLEP) combined with transurethral tissue morcellation: An update on the early clinical experience. Journal of Endourology. 1998;**12**(5):457-459

[11] Ignat M et al. A cost analysis of healthcare episodes including day-case bariatric surgery (roux-en-Y gastric bypass and sleeve gastrectomy) versus inpatient surgery. Obesity Surgery. 2022;**32**(8):2504-2511

[12] Broe M et al. Assessment of routine same-day discharge surgery for robot-assisted radical prostatectomy. World Journal of Urology. 2023;**41**(10):2679-2684

[13] Shvero A et al. HoLEP: The new gold standard for surgical treatment of benign prostatic hyperplasia. The Canadian Journal of Urology. 2021;**28**(S2):6-10

[14] Lokeshwar SD et al. Epidemiology and treatment modalities for the management of benign prostatic hyperplasia. Translational Andrology and Urology. 2019;**8**(5):529

[15] Patel RM, Bariol S. National trends in surgical therapy for benign prostatic

hyperplasia in Australia. ANZ Journal of Surgery. 2019;**89**(4):345-349

[16] Frieben RW et al. The impact of minimally invasive surgeries for the treatment of symptomatic benign prostatic hyperplasia on male sexual function: A systematic review. Asian Journal of Andrology. 2010;**12**(4):500

[17] Malaeb BS et al. National trends in surgical therapy for benign prostatic hyperplasia in the United States (2000-2008). Urology. 2012;**79**(5):1111-1117

[18] Dogan S, Yildiz KY. Our clinic's first experience with HoLEP. Northern Clinics of İstanbul. 2019;**6**(4):355-360

[19] Eaton SH, et al. Cost Analysis of Surgical Approaches Performed by Residents for Bladder Outlet Obstruction: Laser Versus Loop. Open Journal of Urology. 2012;**2**:33-37

[20] Shigemura K et al. Comparison of predictive factors for postoperative incontinence of holmium laser enucleation of the prostate by the surgeons' experience during learning curve. International Neurourology Journal. 2016;**20**(1):59

[21] Bright E, Abrams P. Diseases of the prostate. Reviews in Clinical Gerontology. 2010;**20**(1):10-19

[22] Gilling PJ et al. Long-term results of a randomized trial comparing holmium laser enucleation of the prostate and transurethral resection of the prostate: Results at 7 years. BJU International. 2012;**109**(3):408-411

[23] Erman A et al. Pharmacotherapy vs surgery as initial therapy for patients with moderate-to-severe benign prostate hyperplasia: A cost-effectiveness analysis. BJU International. 2018;**122**(5):879-888

[24] Aladesuru O et al. Review of the economics of surgical treatment options for benign prostatic hyperplasia. Current Urology Reports. 2022;**23**(1):11-18

Chapter 5

Transperineal Laser Ablation of Prostate (TPLA™)

Francesco Sessa, Paolo Polverino and Luisa Moscardi

Abstract

This chapter provides a comprehensive overview of Transperineal Laser Ablation of the prostate (TPLA™) as a therapeutic option for Benign Prostatic Hyperplasia (BPH). BPH is a prevalent condition among aging men, characterized by non-cancerous enlargement of the prostate gland, leading to lower urinary tract symptoms (LUTS) and impacting quality of life. TPLA™ emerges as a minimally invasive technique leveraging the precision of laser energy to induce coagulative necrosis in targeted prostatic tissue, thereby reducing prostate volume and alleviating symptoms. The chapter systematically reviews the procedural aspects of TPLA™, including patient selection criteria, preoperative preparation, and step-by-step surgical technique. Clinical outcomes are discussed, with a focus on symptom relief, improvement in urinary flow rates, and reduction in prostate volume. Furthermore, the safety profile of TPLA™ is examined, documenting the incidence and management of potential complications. In conclusion, TPLA™ represents a promising addition to the therapeutic armamentarium for BPH, offering a balance of efficacy and safety, ensuring high rates of preservation of sexual function.

Keywords: BPH, minimally invasive surgery, LUTS, ejaculation sparing, laser, transperineal laser ablation, TPLA™

1. Introduction

Despite the technological progress achieved in standard surgical techniques for benign prostatic obstruction (BPO), they are still not devoid of side effects and require general or spinal anesthesia as well as hospitalization. Recently, several ultra-minimally invasive surgical techniques were developed with the main goal of finding a compromise between efficacy on urinary symptoms and ejaculation [1]. However, an expanded role of these novel ultra-minimally invasive techniques could be in the setting of highly comorbid patients, potentially not eligible for more invasive surgical procedures [2]. In this view, transperineal laser ablation (TPLA™) of prostate adenoma has shown promising results on efficacy, safety, and impact on sexual function, being feasible in an outpatient setting and using local anesthesia [3]. While the procedure boasts numerous advantages, from the available scientific evidence, a lack of standardization emerges concerning patient selection, treatment execution modalities, intraoperative features, postoperative management, and follow-up [4].

2. Diode laser

The word laser is acronymous for "light amplification by stimulated emission of radiation." Laser light is generated by an energized material (e.g., gas and crystal), and after being absorbed by a tissue, it is converted into thermal energy.

The laser energy has specific features that ensure predictable and precise results. The laser radiation is collimated, coherent, and monochromatic. The term collimated means that the beam travels in only one direction, allowing the laser light to easily enter in very thin flexible optic fibers. The laser energy is defined as coherent because all the photons are emitted at the same time with the same phase, allowing it to reach high energy levels in a short time. Lastly, the laser beam is composed of a single wavelength; it provides specific and selective interaction with tissue chromophores, for this reason it is called monochromatic.

TPLA™ is a modern surgical technique that exploits the benefits of a diode laser to obtain the ablation of prostate adenoma.

2.1 Technical features

In case of diode lasers, the radiation is obtained by a semiconductor-based generator. Depending on wavelengths, commercial lasers emit light in a frequency range of 375–1800 nm. TPLA™ adopts a diode laser with a wavelength of 1064 nm. This wavelength ensures an optimal laser ablation and lower absorption coefficient, which allows the best light penetration into tissues. The specific and selective interaction with the tissue results in a micro-invasive and organ-sparing treatment.

2.2 Biological effect

When the diode laser energy is absorbed by the prostatic tissue, the local temperature increases.

This heating starts to damage the cells until a coagulative necrosis is induced. This phenomenon begins after reaching 60°C inside the tissue, the temperature at which denaturation of proteins begins. As a result, the alteration caused by the laser determines the genesis of a necrotic area that, after an initial inflammatory response, is naturally reorganized by the body hesitating in a scar zone. The maximum extension of the necrosis area is found 72 hours after treatment. Cell damage due to hyperthermia and the occlusion of small and medium-sized blood vessels persist during the days after. For these reasons, the effects of treatment are not immediate, as it takes a few days before starting the cytoreduction process. During the 4–8 weeks after treatment, the scarring processes will be completed with a consequent volume reduction of prostatic gland and urethra decompression.

3. Echolaser system

To date, the only system available to perform transperineal laser ablation of the prostate is the EchoLaser™ (Elesta SpA, Calenzano, Italy). The system consists in two different units – a multisource diode laser generator and the Echolaser Smart Interface – that need to be connected with an ultrasound biplanar probe to plan and execute the ablation.

3.1 Laser generator

The multisource laser generator is composed of four different and independent channels for fiber connection. Each of the four channels is entirely independent of the others; hence, they can be set to different power levels, and it is possible to suspend the laser energy delivery from one or more channels without interrupting the others. Each channel can be connected to a 300-micron optical fiber, enabling the delivery of a variable amount of energy up to a maximum of 6000 J per fiber. The delivery power can be modulated up to a maximum of 7 W (**Figure 1**).

3.2 Echolaser smart interface

The second module of the Echolaser system consists of the Echolaser Smart Interface (ESI), an interface that allows for treatment planning based on the

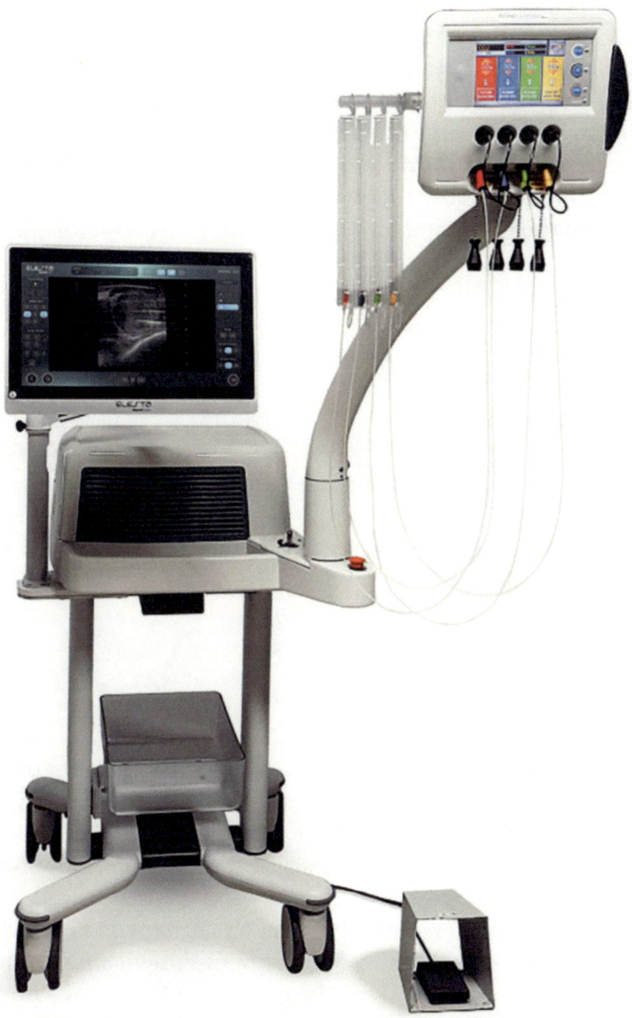

Figure 1.
The Echolaser system with laser generator and the ESI system monitor.

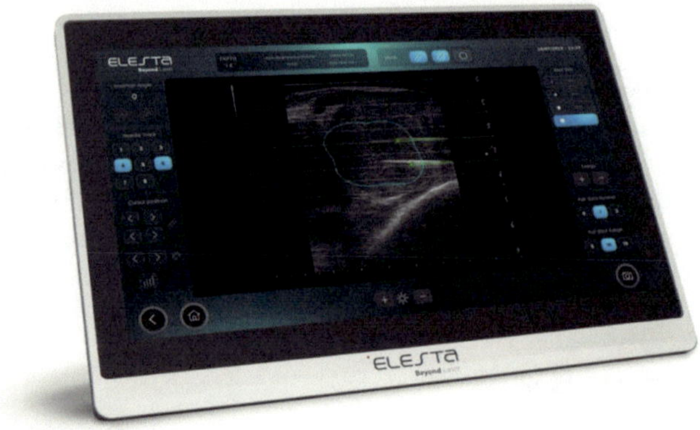

Figure 2.
The Echolaser smart interface (ESI).

morphological characteristics of the prostate and guides the positioning of the laser fibers. Echolaser Smart Interface (ESI) technology allows the visualization of needles trajectories during their insertion. ESI overlaps on the US image a cyan area where critical structures should not be contained. This area is designed by changing different parameters to best fit the volume and shape of the prostate adenoma (**Figure 2**).

This dedicated simulation software helps the user to plan the treatment, facilitating the assessment of the following parameters:

- Insertion angle
- Number and position of needles
- Mutual needle position
- Different energy levels (to be set by the user)
- Number of pull-backs (if needed, see the dedicated paragraph 6.4)
- Distance of pull-back

4. Patient selection

TPLA™ is an ultra-minimally invasive option for the treatment of lower urinary tract symptoms (LUTS) due to benign prostatic obstruction (BPO). Despite the increasing utilization of this technique, as of today, it has not been included in the recommendations of international guidelines, and there is no standardization in patient selection.

In terms of dimensions, an essential prerequisite for adequate ablation is a prostatic volume > 30 ml; nevertheless, there is no upper dimensional limit from a technical standpoint. Some authors discourage the procedure in case of a large median lobe (>1.5 cm); however, opinions in the literature are divergent [3]. TPLA™ should be avoided in cases of urethral stenosis, bladder neck contracture, prior prostate surgery, and severe reduction in bladder contractility. The presence of an indwelling catheter is not a contraindication to treatment. The presence of anal stenosis might pose difficulty in performing the treatment due to the requirement of positioning a transrectal ultrasound probe.

The procedure represents a valid option for patients with moderate to severe urinary symptoms, who are motivated to preserve ejaculation, unable to tolerate medical therapy, or deemed unfit for traditional surgery due to high anesthesiologic or perioperative risk.

5. Preoperative preparation

The TPLA™ is a simple and quick procedure; however, a meticulous preparation of equipment and operating settings is suggested to facilitate its execution.

5.1 Preliminary assessment

For a comprehensive preparatory assessment of the patient, it is advisable to collect routine blood testing and functional questionnaires (The International Prostate Symptom Score, IPSS; the International Index of Erectile Function, IIEF-5; Male Sexual Health Questionnaire-Ejaculatory Dysfunction Short Form, MSHQ-EjD SF) and non-invasive urodynamics data (maximum flow rate, Qmax; post-void residual, PVR) [4].

In patients taking antiplatelet or anticoagulant medications, discontinuation of these drugs should be evaluated on a case-by-case basis; however, it is not mandatory for the execution of the treatment.

5.2 Medical equipment and operative setting

The procedure can be performed in an outpatient setting equipped with an examination table featuring dedicated leg supports. The availability of a biplanar ultrasound probe is a necessary condition for performing the treatment. A sterile field with all necessary equipment for the procedure will be set up on a serving trolley:

- 3-way 18Ch catheter
- Antiseptic for skin disinfection (e.g., povidone iodine)
- Lidocaine
- Syringe and needles for subcutaneous anesthesia and periprostatic block
- Introducer needles (21G Chiba needles)
- Optical fibers: 300 μm quartz
- Sterile drapes

5.3 Patient positioning

The patient is placed in the lithotomy position on leg supports. A three-way 18-F Foley catheter is placed with continuous irrigation to ensure cooling of the urethral wall during lasing time, avoiding possible thermal damage. Subsequently, the perineum is exposed using adhesive tapes, and the sterile surgical field is prepared.

5.4 Antibiotic and antithrombotic prophylaxis

To reduce perioperative infectious risk, it is advisable to prescribe antibiotic prophylaxis. Perioperative intravenous single shot of 2 g cephazolin is administrated within 1 hour before the procedure. Medical thromboprophylaxis is usually not required.

5.5 Anesthesia

One of the primary advantages of this technique is the feasibility to be performed under local anesthesia, optionally combined with conscious sedation. The method of performing local anesthesia is similar to that used for transperineal prostate biopsies: initial anesthesia of the perineal skin is followed by a periprostatic block. The recommended dosage of anesthetic is approximately 30 ml of 1% lidocaine. According to patients' preference, it's possible to administer oral benzodiazepines or intravenous midazolam for conscious sedation.

The decision to perform the procedure under local anesthesia ensures greater speed of execution, the ability to treat patients with high anesthetic risk, and the use of an outpatient setting, resulting in economic and organizational advantages. However, based on operating room availability and/or patient and operator preferences, the procedure may also be performed under spinal or general anesthesia.

6. Surgical technique: transperineal laser ablation of prostate adenoma

Two distinct phases of the surgical procedure can be identified: fiber placement and laser ablation. The successful outcome of the treatment relies on meticulous preoperative planning.

6.1 Transrectal ultrasound and surgical planning

After setting up the surgical field with appropriate sterile draping, the biplanar ultrasound probe for transrectal ultrasound is introduced. At this point, the periprostatic block is performed by injecting approximately 15–20 ml of 1% lidocaine posteriorly, laterally, and anteriorly to the prostatic capsule. Subsequently, measurements of prostate and prostatic adenoma dimensions are taken. Depending on the morphology and size of the gland, the treatment will be planned with the ESI system. Using ESI, the intended treatment area will be visualized, with larger volumes as the delivered energy increases, up to a maximum of 1800 J per fiber. In the case of large prostates, if it is necessary to expand the treatment area, it is possible to plan an ablation with two fibers per lobe and/or plan a pull-back for the treatment of the apical portion of the adenoma. For each fiber, it is possible to set different ablation areas, different pull-back lengths, and visualize the intended treatment areas both in sagittal and axial view (**Figure 3**).

6.2 Needles and fibers positioning

In light of the planned ablation, the introducer needles are positioned, readily available in the kit provided by the manufacturer. These consist of a 21G Chiba

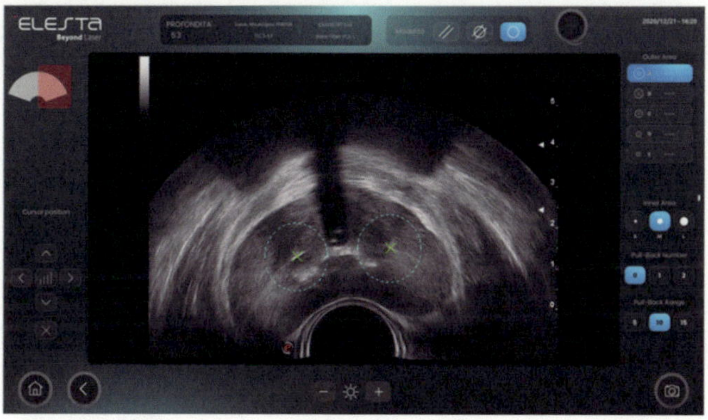

Figure 3.
Surgical planning with ESI system. The cyan area represents the virtual extension of the ablation.

needle, which also features a stopper to secure it in place once the desired position is reached. The needles can be inserted either with a dedicated needle guide or freehand, depending on the operator's preference and experience in transperineal approach. After inserting the introducer needle, it is crucial to verify that safety distances are respected in the axial plane. The needle tip, visualized ultrasonographically as a hyperechoic point, should be at least 8 mm away from the urethra and the prostatic capsule bilaterally. At this stage, the ESI system simulation comes to aid once again, displaying a cyan circular area with the needle at its center, showing the hypothetical treatment area with the safety distances already respected. When two needles are placed per lobe, the minimum distance to maintain between each needle is 5 mm.

Next, the stylets of the Chiba needles are removed, and the optical fibers are inserted. These fibers extend 10 mm beyond the needle tip, which is why safety distances in the sagittal plane with the bladder neck need to be checked only after their insertion; the bladder neck should be at least 15 mm away from the fiber tip. Once again, the ESI system can be utilized at this stage. Once the final position of the needle-fiber system is established, it can be secured using the stopper (**Figures 4–6**).

6.3 Ablation settings

The laser fiber consists of an energy delivery tip and a connector that must be connected to the generator. Before proceeding with the insertion of the laser fiber into the needle, it is advisable to verify its proper functioning. Upon activation, it emits a flashing red circle.

There is no standardization regarding the energy delivery mode. The generator allows for energy delivery with variable power ranging from 0 to 7 W. Typically, it is advisable to start the ablation with a power of 5 W and potentially reduce it to 3 W in case of discomfort or intense burning sensation reported by the patient. In case the procedure is performed in the operating room under spinal or general anesthesia, it is possible to execute the entire procedure with a maximum power delivery of 7 W.

The ablation is initiated by the operator using a dedicated pedal, which allows for interruption of the procedure at any time. As soon as the energy delivery begins, it is advisable to gently move the fibers to facilitate ignition. The ablative effect will manifest ultrasonographically as the formation of hyperechoic bubbles (*bubbling effect*) (**Figures 7** and **8**).

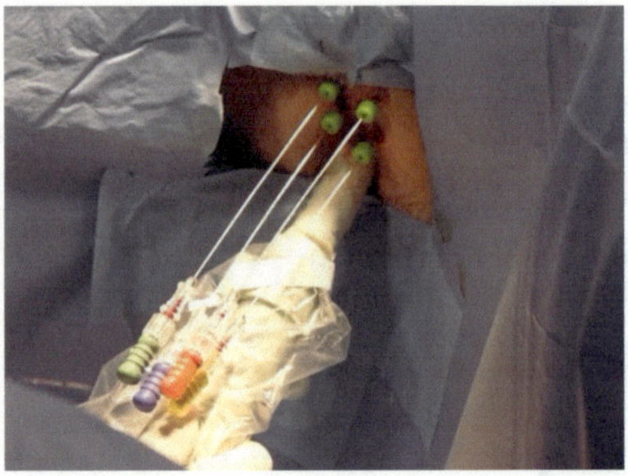

Figure 4.
Treatment with two needles per lobe. Fibers position in the perineum skin.

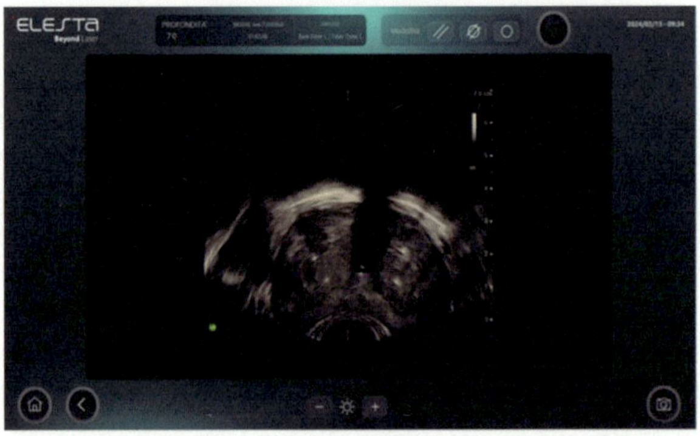

Figure 5.
Treatment with two needles per lobe. Fibers position in the prostate at transrectal ultrasound.

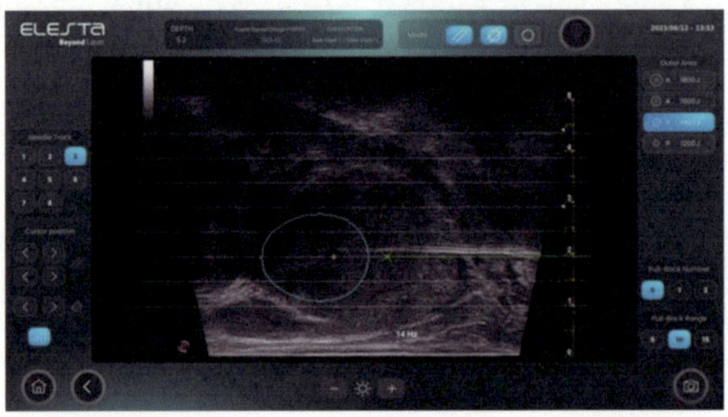

Figure 6.
Longitudinal view after fiber insertion. The fiber tip goes 10 mm ahead of the needle tip. The distance from bladder neck must be checked after fiber insertion.

6.4 Pull-back technique

As described in the preceding paragraphs, the maximum area that can be treated corresponds to a delivery of 1800 J. The effect of the delivered energy indeed reaches a plateau volume at this threshold: giving more than 1800 J in a single illumination will not

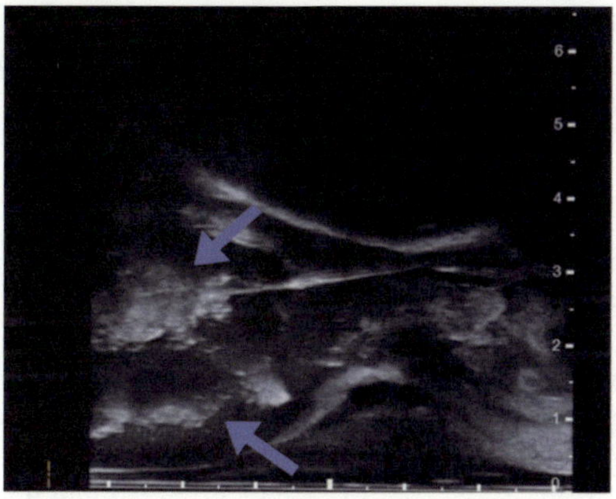

Figure 7.
Hyperechoic bubbling effect during laser ablation, longitudinal view.

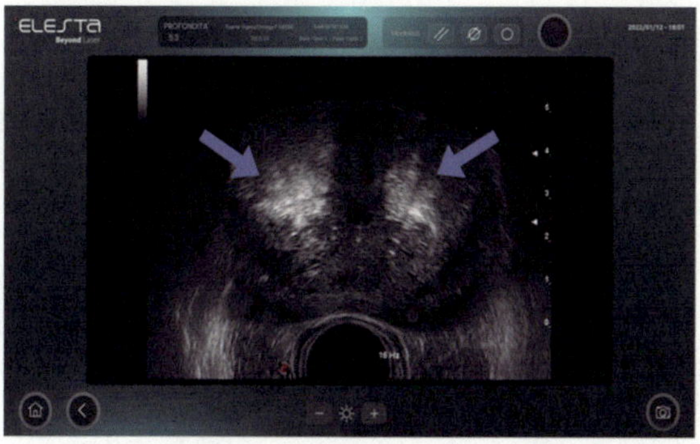

Figure 8.
Hyperechoic bubbling effect during laser ablation, axial view.

increase the treated volume. Therefore, to achieve a larger treated area, two alternatives are possible: increase the number of positioned fibers and/or perform a new ablation by retracting the fiber itself into the most apical portion of the adenoma. This latter method is called the pull-back technique. It involves a second ablation performed after retracting the fiber by 5–10 mm. Its execution can be planned in advance with the ESI system, which is crucial for those who are new to the technique. Often, the hyperechoic effect generated by the treatment makes it difficult to identify the fiber within the prostatic parenchyma after the first ablation. For this reason, it is possible to determine the retraction distance using the graduated notches positioned on the needle and spaced 10 mm apart.

After the fiber retraction, a second ablation is performed. Once again, it is possible to deliver energy ranging from 1200 to 1800 J depending on the volume to be treated. The overall duration of the treatment varies according to the delivered energy, power, and number of pull-backs; for a prostate of average size (approximately 60 ml), it ranges from 5 to 10 minutes.

6.5 Technical nuances

The transperineal laser ablation of prostate adenoma stands at the forefront of minimally invasive interventions for managing benign prostatic hyperplasia. As an innovative technique, mastering the nuances and optimizing procedural efficacy are paramount for medical professionals engaged in its practice. Below are some technical suggestions and tips to enhance the operator's technical skills and improve the outcome of the procedure.

- High-volume prostates: In case of prostatic volume > 60–70 ml consider positioning four fibers (two fibers for lobe) and performing a second ablation using the pull-back technique;

- Asymmetric lobes: In case of asymmetric lobes, consider positioning three fibers and/or delivering different amounts of energy to the two lobes;

- Prostatic calcifications and cysts: In case of prostatic calcification and cysts, place the fiber tip a few millimeters away from it to allow the propagation of the laser energy;

- Needle guidance: Using needle guidance may be very useful during the first procedures or in case of low experience with the transperineal approach. The freehand needle positioning ensures more dexterity and flexibility, allowing the place of the fiber into the exact desired point and potentially adjusting the insertion angle to reach certain parts of the adenoma (e.g., in cases of prostates with greater anteroposterior development, the anterior part of the adenoma may be difficult to reach due to the presence of the pubis);

- Evaluation of hyperechogenicity effect: during the ablation, the treatment effect is ultrasonographically translated into a hyperechoic signal. However, its extent does not accurately reflect the actual ablation size. For these reasons, it is crucial for the operator not to be influenced by this ultrasound artifact but to always rely on the preparatory planning carried out beforehand with the ESI system.

7. Postoperative management

After the treatment, the clinical effect is not immediate. The process from coagulative necrosis to complete absorption of the ablated tissue requires a period ranging from 4 to 8 weeks. Consequently, the clinical benefits are not direct but follow the course of the cytoreductive process.

In the postoperative period, ensuring good clinical outcomes relies heavily on proper therapeutic management and tailoring choices to the patient's characteristics and the treatment performed.

7.1 Catheter removal

The timing of urinary catheter removal in patients undergoing TPLA™ is one of the most debated topics in the literature. Some authors advocate for immediate removal of the urinary catheter at the end of the treatment, while it is common practice to wait 5–7 days before proceeding with catheter removal [3, 4].

This allows for an initial reduction of edema that develops following the treatment, which could have a 'paradoxical effect,' resulting in an increased risk of urinary retention. In particular clinical conditions, such as in the case of catheters carriers, history of urinary retention or in case of a high amount of delivery energy the catheter may be left in place for a longer period (up to 2 weeks). On the other hand, in young patients, not strongly obstructed, with medium to small-sized prostates, it may be possible to attempt catheter removal at the end of the treatment and await subsequent resumption of spontaneous micturition.

7.2 Medical therapy

After catheter removal, the patient may also experience urinary symptoms consistent with the inflammatory process underway. Particularly common symptoms include frequent urination, urgency, and dysuria. In this phase, it is important to manage inflammatory symptoms with appropriate pharmacological support. This ensures symptom relief and simultaneous reduction of the infectious risk associated with the procedure.

A common choice is to administer antibiotics and anti-inflammatory drugs for at least 7–10 days, and in some cases to continue BPH therapy for 1 month. In detail, a possible therapeutic regimen is as follows:

- Low dose Corticosteroids: Methylprednisolone for 10 days (in case of severe diabetes: Ibuprofen 600 mg bid for 7 days);
- Antibiotics: Cefixime 400 mg daily for 5 days;
- Alpha blockers: e.g. Alfuzosin for 20 days;
- NSAIDs: e.g. Ibuprofen 600 mg on demand in case of pain.

8. Complications

Transperineal laser ablation (TPLA™) has emerged as a minimally invasive treatment option for benign prostatic hyperplasia (BPH), offering promising outcomes with reduced morbidity compared to traditional surgical approaches. However, like any medical intervention, TPLA™ is associated with potential complications that necessitate thorough understanding and management. In the literature, the overall complication rate ranged from 0 to 13%, and there were mostly early complications within 30 days of treatment [3].

Below are listed the possible complications:

- Urinary retention: Either acute or delayed, it can occur following TPLA™ due to post-procedural edema or prostatic swelling. Patients should be monitored closely after catheter removal, and urinary catheterization may be required to relieve obstruction;
- Hematuria: It can occur more frequently in patients taking antiplatelets or anticoagulants. It is usually mild, and it typically resolves spontaneously within a few days. However, in case of severe or persistent hematuria may necessitate intervention, including bladder irrigation or clot evacuation;

- Urinary tract infections (UTIs): UTIs are potential complications of TPLA™. Prophylactic antibiotics are administered perioperatively to reduce the risk of UTIs and are typically continued for 5–7 days after the procedure;

- Prostatic abscess: It is a very rare complication, with an incidence ranging from 0 to 5% of cases in the literature. The formation of a prostatic abscess occurs due to bacterial proliferation in the tissue cavitation generated by laser ablation. It is treated with antibiotic therapy and percutaneous ultrasound-guided drainage;

- Ejaculatory dysfunction: TPLA™ may result in ejaculatory dysfunction, characterized by reduced ejaculate volume or retrograde ejaculation. Preservation of ejaculatory function depends on the extent of tissue ablation and proximity to the ejaculatory ducts. Its rate of incidence ranges from 0 to 4%;

- Erectile dysfunction, urethral stricture, and incontinence: These are extremely rare adverse effects if the treatment is performed while adhering to the safety distances described in the preceding paragraphs.

9. Results

Studies evaluating the efficacy of TPLA™ consistently report significant improvements in LUTS scores following the procedure [5]. Reductions in International Prostate Symptom Score (IPSS) and improvement in quality of life (QoL) metrics are commonly observed within weeks to months post-TPLA™. Long-term follow-up studies demonstrate sustained symptom relief, with many patients experiencing durable benefits over several years [6, 7]. This is also reflected in the urodynamic parameters: TPLA™ effectively improves urodynamic parameters associated with BPH, including increased urinary flow rates and reduced post-void residual volume. These improvements correlate with symptomatic relief and contribute to enhanced urinary function and patient satisfaction. From a safety standpoint as well, it has been demonstrated that the procedure is safe with a very low risk of adverse events. Additionally, TPLA™ can be performed under local anesthesia, reducing the risks associated with general anesthesia and facilitating outpatient procedures. In this regard, a recent study evaluated the outcomes of this technique in a population of multi-morbid and high-risk patients, confirming its safety and efficacy even in this subset of patients [2]. If compared to the current gold standard therapy represented by transurethral resection of the prostate (TURP), the risk of sexual and ejaculatory dysfunctions is significantly lower, with a lower increase of the Qmax values but a similar impact on urinary symptoms evaluated by the IPSS questionnaire, as demonstrated by two RCTs [8, 9].

10. Conclusion

In conclusion, TPLA™ emerges as a promising minimally invasive technique for the treatment of Benign Prostatic Obstruction. Through the application of laser energy, TPLA™ offers a targeted and tailored approach to address the enlarged prostate tissue, providing relief from bothersome lower urinary tract symptoms while preserving sexual function and minimizing complications.

TPLA™'s efficacy in reducing prostate volume and improving urinary flow parameters has been demonstrated in numerous clinical studies. Furthermore, the transperineal approach offers advantages over transurethral procedures by reducing the risk of complications such as urethral strictures, urinary incontinence, and sexual dysfunction. This approach also allows for precise targeting of prostate tissue, minimizing damage to surrounding structures and promoting quicker recovery times.

The aforementioned characteristics make the technique appealing to younger patients, who are strongly interested in preserving ejaculatory function. However, it is also safely applicable to elderly, frail patients with multiple comorbidities, who would otherwise be excluded from any other surgical therapeutic option.

The technique also presents advantages from an economic and management perspective: the possibility of performing it in an outpatient setting and under local anesthesia drastically reduces the costs related to hospitalization and operating room utilization. From a public health perspective, it may help to reduce waiting times for surgery.

Conflict of interest

The authors declare no conflict of interest.

Author details

Francesco Sessa*, Paolo Polverino and Luisa Moscardi
Unit of Urological Robotic Surgery and Renal Transplantation, Careggi Hospital, University of Florence, Florence, Italy

*Address all correspondence to: francesco_sessa@hotmail.it

IntechOpen

© 2024 The Author(s). Licensee IntechOpen. This chapter is distributed under the terms of the Creative Commons Attribution License (http://creativecommons.org/licenses/by/4.0), which permits unrestricted use, distribution, and reproduction in any medium, provided the original work is properly cited.

References

[1] Checcucci E, Veccia A, De Cillis S, Piramide F, Volpi G, Amparore D, et al. Uro-technology and SoMe working group of the young academic urologists working party of the European Association of Urology and of the Lower Tract and Research Group of the European Section of Uro-technology. New ultra-minimally invasive surgical treatment for benign prostatic hyperplasia: A systematic review and analysis of comparative outcomes. European Urology Open Science. 2021;**33**:28-41

[2] Polverino P, Lo Re M, Saladino M, Pecoraro A, Moscardi L, Rivetti A, et al. Could transperineal interstitial laser ablation of the prostate be the right option for highly-comorbid patients with lower urinary tract symptoms due to benign prostatic obstruction? A preliminary single-center experience focusing on functional and safety outcomes. Minerva Urology and Nephrology. 2023. DOI: 10.23736/S2724-6051.23.05479-4. [Epub ahead of print]

[3] Sessa F, Polverino P, Siena G, Bisegna C, Lo Re M, Spatafora P, et al. Transperineal laser ablation of the prostate (TPLA) for lower urinary tract symptoms due to benign prostatic obstruction. Journal of Clinical Medicine. 2023;**12**(3):793. DOI: 10.3390/jcm12030793

[4] Pacella CM, Patelli G, Iapicca G, Manenti G, Perretta T, Ryan CP, et al. Transperineal laser ablation for percutaneous treatment of benign prostatic hyperplasia: A feasibility study. Results at 6 and 12 months from a retrospective multi-centric study. Prostate Cancer and Prostatic Diseases. 2020;**23**:356-363

[5] Tafuri A, Panunzio A, De Carlo F, Luperto E, Di Cosmo F, Cavaliere A, et al. Transperineal laser ablation for benign prostatic enlargement: A systematic review and pooled analysis of pilot studies. Journal of Clinical Medicine. 2023;**12**(5):1860. DOI: 10.3390/jcm12051860

[6] Patelli G, Altieri VM, Ierardi AM, Carnevale A, Chizzoli F, Baronchelli G, et al. Transperineal laser ablation of the prostate for symptomatic benign prostatic hyperplasia: Long-term follow-up in 40 patients. Journal of Vascular and Interventional Radiology. 2024:S1051-0443(24)00326-9. DOI: 10.1016/j.jvir.2024.04.023. [Epub ahead of print]

[7] Minafra P, Rienzo GDE, Gerbasi S, Cindolo L, Battaglia M, Ditonno P. Three years outcomes of transperineal laser ablation of the prostate. Minerva Urology and Nephrology. 2023;**75**(4):471-478. DOI: 10.23736/S2724-6051.23.05270-9. Epub 2023 June 14

[8] Bertolo R, Iacovelli V, Cipriani C, Carilli M, Vittori M, Antonucci M, et al. Ejaculatory function following transperineal laser ablation vs TURP for benign prostatic obstruction: A randomized trial. BJU International. 2023;**132**(1):100-108. DOI: 10.1111/bju.16008. Epub 2023 March 30

[9] Canat HL, Gurbuz C, Bozkurt M. Transurethral resection of the prostate (TURP) versus transperineal laser ablation (TPLA) due to benign prostatic hyperplasia (BPH): Prospective and comparative study. International Urology and Nephrology. 2023;**55**(11):2747-2752. DOI: 10.1007/s11255-023-03717-8. Epub 2023 July 27

Chapter 6

Benign Prostatic Hyperplasia and Its Effect on Male Infertility

Julius Akhaine and Ifiok Umana

Abstract

Benign prostatic hyperplasia (BPH) is known to negatively impact male fertility. This can occur via various mechanisms. It can be due to the intrinsic enlargement of the prostate gland, inflammation of the prostate gland and its contiguous structures, as well as the treatment modalities of BPH. Most of the treatment options for LUTS due to BPH, both pharmacologic and surgical, are known to have significant sexual side effects and most importantly ejaculatory dysfunction. While ejaculatory dysfunction due to pharmacologic therapy is usually reversible on cessation of treatment, that attributable to surgical interventions is often permanent and irreversible. Some medications has been shown to directly or indirectly improve sperm parameters such as sperm count and concentration, motility, as well as morphology. Hormone mediating agents such as clomiphene citrate and antioxidant based supplements such as vitamins C, E, and D, as well as zinc and coenzyme Q10 have found a common use by most urologists. Some novel therapies are now used to treat BPH in a bid to mitigate the problem of infertility associated with common conventional treatment options and thus enhance the chances of spouse conception in these affected men, and a notable example today is the Urolift.

Keywords: BPH, male infertility, erectile dysfunction, LUTS, semen, TURP

1. Introduction

1.1 Definition of benign prostatic hyperplasia (BPH)

Benign prostatic hyperplasia (BPH) is a common pathologic condition that affect men mostly in their midlife. It is the main cause of lower urinary tract symptoms in older men [1]. It is also one of the factors associated with male infertility; although BPH in itself may not directly cause male infertility, it can lead to certain complications that may influence fertility [2].

BPH can be described as a pathologic condition characterised by the proliferation of the cellular elements of the prostate with a resultant glandular enlargement. This enlargement involves both the stromal and epithelial components of the prostate or an impairment of programmed cell death causing cellular accumulation [3].

1.2 Anatomy and physiology of the prostate gland

The prostate gland is a fibro-muscular glandular organ located within the male pelvis behind the pubic symphysis, from which it is separated by the pubo-prostatic ligaments, fibro-fatty tissue, and blood vessels. The normal prostate resembles an inverted pyramid and measures 3–4 cm at the base, 4–6 cm in cephalo-caudal, and 2–3 cm in antero-posterior dimensions, and weighs 18–26 g. It has an apex, the inferior limit, and a base on which the bladder rests. Throughout its length run the urethra and ejaculatory ducts. Related structures include the rectum and Denonvilliers fascia that lie posterior to the prostate and paired seminal vesicles and ampullae of the vasa deferentia that lie postero-lateral to the prostate and posterior to the bladder [4].

Embryologically, it starts to develop by the 12th week of gestation under the influence of testosterone from the testes of the developing foetus. It develops from the urogenital sinus through dihydrotestosterone (DHT) stimulation. The primary motivation behind prostate development is androgen receptor signalling through DHT, which is diffusely found in the entire genito-urinary tract. The prostate originates from epithelial buds formed at precise locations via mechanisms that are still not fully understood under the influence of paralogous homeobox (Hox) genes, fibroblast growth factor (FGF) family, transforming growth factor-β subfamily etc. [5].

The prostatic epithelium is composed of two major cellular compartments: epithelial and stromal. The prostate epithelial compartment consists of basal epithelial cells, intermediate cells, neuro-endocrine cells, and luminal secretory cells while the stromal compartment consists mainly of connective tissue, smooth muscle cells, and fibroblast and serves to provide structural support.

The seminal plasma is formed primarily from secretions of the sex accessory tissues, which provide suitable milieu for survival and function of spermatozoa. The prostate provides about 0.5 ml to the estimated 2–6 ml of normal ejaculate. The secretion of the prostate consist mainly of prostate specific antigen (PSA, human kallikrein-3) human kallikrein-2, prostase, prostate acid phosphatase (PAP) and prostate specific protein (PSP-94). These prostatic secretions are believed to play key roles in regulation of semen coagulation and liquefaction [5].

1.3 Prevalence and incidence of BPH

BPH being a disease condition associated with ageing is associated with varying prevalence and incidence. A landmark study by Berry et al. in 1984 demonstrated that no men younger than 30 years of age had evidence of BPH and that the prevalence rose with each age group, peaking at 88% in men in their 80s [3]. As world health systems are improving with associated higher life expectancy, the incidence and prevalence of BPH have also increased rapidly [6]. Lee et al. in their meta-analysis found that the lifetime prevalence of BPH worldwide was 26.2% (95% CI: 22.8–29.6%) and their results that nearly 1 in 4 men will suffer from BPH over their lifetime [7]. There were about 94.0 million (95% UI: 73.2–118.0) prevalent cases of BPH worldwide in 2019, compared with 51.1 million (95% UI: 43.1–69.3) cases in 2000. This shows a sharp rise in the prevalence of BPH, and this was particularly noticed in the low-income and middle-income countries that are presently undergoing rapid demographic and epidemiological changes [8].

DOI: http://dx.doi.org/10.5772/intechopen.1006156

1.4 Definition of male infertility

The World Health Organisation in its 2024 edition of the International Classification of Diseases (ICD-11) defined infertility as a disease of the reproductive system defined by the failure to achieve a clinical pregnancy after 12 months or more of regular, unprotected sexual intercourse [9]. This definition applies to both males and females. However, the male factor has been cited to contribute about 50% to infertility in many studies [10].

2. Overview of BPH

2.1 Causes and risk factors of BPH

The causes or aetiology of BPH remains uncertain; however, multiple theories have been propounded to explain it. Advanced age and androgen are two strong risk factors associated with BPH. Several mechanisms seem to be at work in the pathogenesis and progression of BPH, some of which are listed below.

The figure below shows a complex interplay of several factors all culminating in inflammation, which serves as the final pathway to the development of BPH (**Figure 1**).

2.1.1 Sex hormones

2.1.1.1 Androgens

The role of androgens in the development of BPH has been widely published. Androgen Receptor (AR) may lead to the development of BPH via epithelial cell-stromal interaction with the alterations of epithelial-mesenchymal transition, thus bringing about stromal cell proliferation. The serum testosterone levels may be lower in ageing men when compared with healthy younger men; however, the levels of dihydrotestosterone (DHT) are elevated. Thus, patients with BPH have significant higher

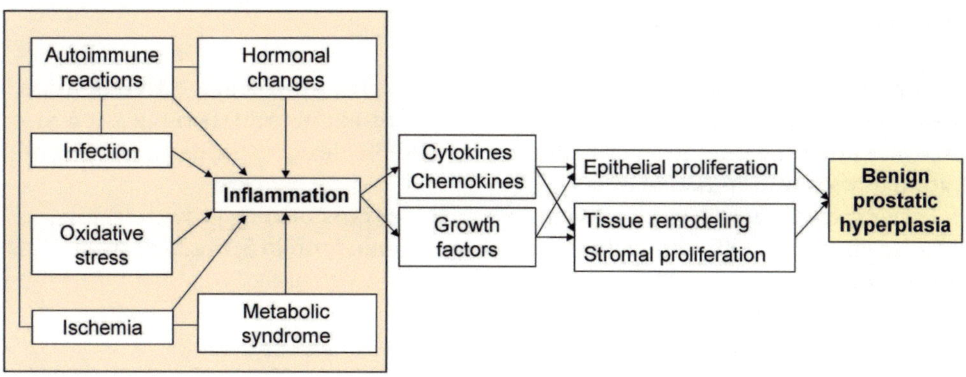

Figure 1.
Factors associated with the proliferative process of BPH. Adapted from Ref. [11].

levels of serum DHT than do unaffected men of similar age [12, 13]. This finding underlies the principle of the use of 5-α reductase inhibitors in the treatment of BPH, suggesting an up-regulation of the enzyme in men with BPH.

2.1.1.2 Oestrogens

Serum oestrogens do not display an age-related change like serum androgens. Oestrogen has been implicated in the proliferation of prostatic stromal cells. The activation of oestrogen receptors expressed in the prostate gland leads to aberrant proliferation and inflammation of the gland. Robert et al. stated that BPH patients had higher serum oestradiol levels or oestradiol/testosterone ratios [14]. While King et al. reported that normal prostate stromal cell proliferation was stimulated by an increase in the ratio of oestrogen/androgen and also that the proliferation of normal prostatic epithelial cells was stimulated by an indirect action of steroids mediated by stromal cells [15].

Aromatase has also been implicated in the development of BPH. It is reported that the blocking of the conversion of androgens to oestrogens by aromatase inhibitors appears to prevent prostatic hyperplasia [16].

2.1.2 Growth factors

2.1.2.1 Insulin-like growth factor-1

Insulin-like growth factor-1 (IGF-1) is expressed in the stromal and epithelial cells of the prostate. This has been found to be true especially in patients with acromegaly. Kumar et al. reported that these patients have higher prostate volume than healthy controls [17].

2.1.2.2 Fibroblast growth factor

Fibroblast growth factor-2 (FGF-2) is expressed abundantly in the prostate epithelium and stroma. FGF-2 is mitogenic to the prostate and there is an association of FGF-2 with prostate stromal proliferation [18].

2.1.2.3 Epidermal growth factor

Epithelial growth factor (EGF) is associated with the growth and differentiation of epithelial cells in the prostate. It is abundantly present in prostate tissues. It is also discovered that the inhibition of EGF receptor (EGFR) leads to the decreased proliferation of prostatic epithelial cells [19].

Other growth factors implicated in BPH include transforming growth factors, vascular endothelial growth factor, bone morphogenic protein 5, brain-derived neurotrophic factor, thyroid hormones, etc.

2.1.3 Chronic inflammation

BPH is an immunoinflammatory disease [20]. Chronic inflammation has been implicated in the pathogenesis of BPH. Kohnen et al. reported that histologic inflammation was found in 98.1% of patients undergoing transurethral resection of the prostate (TURP) for BPH with lower urinary symptoms (LUTS) [21]. The REDUCE trial gave credence to this postulation when it reported that chronic inflammation was found in 77.6% of prostate biopsy cases and prostate volume was significantly larger in the group with chronic inflammation than in those without it [22].

Some inflammatory mediators involved in the pathogenesis of chronic inflammation in BPH include lymphocytes, monocytes/macrophages, IL-8, IL-17, etc. [23, 24].

2.1.4 Race

Race is an independent risk factor for the development of BPH. It has been reported that Caucasian men are more likely to develop BPH than their African-American counterparts (9.9% vs. 4.1%, respectively); however, surgical interventions meant for severe BPH was more common in African-American men [25]. A study by Hellwege et al. reported that BPH is likely heritable [26].

2.1.5 Microbiota

Several postulations have been made about microbiota contributing to the pathogenesis of prostatic proliferation. The microbiota said to be associated with prostatic enlargement include gut microbiota, urine microbiota, and prostate microbiota.

Takezaka et al. reported that Firmicutes/Bacteroides ratio of gut microbiota was significantly higher in patients with enlarged prostates [27].

The changes in the bladder microbiota might be associated with increasing LUTS in older men. Tsai et al. reported that the urine microbiota composition of patients with BPH was different from those of the control and consisted of Alcaligenes, Pseudomonas, Lactobacillus, Akkermansia, and Cetobacterium [28].

Okada et al. reported that the prostate microbiota were found in the prostatic duct. Isolates from the BPH tissue included *Escherichia coli*, *Staphylococcus*, and *Micrococcus spp*. [29, 30].

2.2 Symptoms and diagnostic methods for BPH

Patients with BPH present with a constellation of symptoms generally referred to as lower urinary tract symptoms (LUTS). These symptom complexes can be grouped as voiding, storage, and post-micturition symptoms. The voiding symptoms include hesitancy, poor stream, intermittency, and straining; the storage symptoms are frequency, urgency, urge incontinence, and nocturia; while the post-micturition symptoms are feeling of incomplete bladder emptying and terminal dribbling. Other symptoms may include haematuria, features of uraemia or urosepsis. Urinary retention, etc. some patients may also experience erectile dysfunction, infertility, as well as a reduction in the quality of life (QoL). The symptoms of BPH can be objectively assessed using validated tools like the International Prostate Symptom Score (IPSS). Scores of 0–7, 8–19, and 20–35 would translate to mild, moderate, and severe symptoms, respectively [31].

Examination findings may reveal features with or without of symptoms. There may be abdominal findings like groin hernias or suprapubic fullness with or without tenderness. A digital rectal examination (DRE) may show features of an enlarged prostate with characteristic features suggestive of BPH like non-tender, firm, smooth, rubbery, non-nodular, preserved median groove and lateral sulci, and examining finger not stained with blood.

The diagnostic methods in diagnosing BPH consist of clinical evaluation using history and physical examination. It is worthy of note to state that the diagnosis of BPH is clinical. However, investigations may be carried out to confirm the diagnosis as well as assess the extent of the disease and plann for the treatment. Definitively, the diagnosis of BPH can be made only with a prostate biopsy and histology.

The investigations would include urinalysis; urine microscopy, culture, and sensitivity; comprehensive metabolic panel (CMP); complete blood count (CBC); prostate-specific antigen (PSA); and urologic ultrasonography (kidneys, ureters, bladder, prostate volume, and postvoid urine residual volume). Baseline urodynamic studies like uroflowmetry can also be done. Retrograde cystoscopy can be carried out when indicated.

2.3 Treatment options for BPH

The treatment options for BPH could be categorized using the IPSS as a guide. Mild symptoms can be treated by conservative modalities, moderate symptoms by medical therapy, and severe symptoms by surgical intervention.

The conservative treatment modalities would include watchful waiting and lifestyle and dietary modifications.

Medical therapy would consist of the use of pharmacological agents like α1-adrenoceptor blockers alone or in combination with 5α-reductase inhibitors, muscarinic receptor antagonists, β-3 agonists, phosphodiesterase 5 inhibitors, and some plant extracts.

The surgical treatment of BPH can be grouped as resection, enucleation, vaporization, alternative ablative techniques, and non-ablative techniques [32].

3. Impact of BPH and BPH-related treatments on infertility

3.1 Effects of BPH on sperm production and semen quality

The precise molecular aetiology of this hyperplastic process is uncertain. The observed increase in cell number may be due to epithelial and stromal proliferation or to impaired programmed cell death leading to cellular accumulation. Multiple factors have been postulated in the aetiology as androgens, estrogens, stromal-epithelial interactions, growth factors, and neurotransmitters may play a role, either singly or in combination, in the aetiology of the hyperplastic process. Also, inflammatory cell infiltrates have been seen in many men with BPH and this may be an additional source of growth factors in human BPH tissue [5, 33].

Taking into account that the prostate gland is the major male accessory gland and has anatomic connection to the testes by way of the vas deferens, its pathology exerts attendant negative effect on essential functions of the male gonad and thereby affects male fertility. The key contribution of prostatic fluid to enhance male fertility is related to its role as a trigger for the molecular pathways involved in ejaculation, sperm activation and capacitation, and more importantly in evoking gene expression, cellular changes, and tissue remodelling in the female reproductive tract and immune system, thus actively influencing fertility and fecundity. A state of local inflammation can alter male fertility either directly by impairing sperm quality or indirectly by causing prostate dysfunction [34].

The mechanical obstruction caused by the enlarged gland and resultant stasis of urine forms a podium for recurrent urinary tract infection, prostatitis, and by extension chronic orchitis, which can affect optimal testicular function, sperm production, and sperm characteristics and function directly. Uropathogens may alter sperm quality through different mechanisms: direct sperm damage, inflammation induced damage, or gland dysfunction. Cumulative evidence indicates that infection and inflammation of the prostate are detrimental to sperm quality and male fertility.

Additionally, some drugs used in the management of BPH and its associated complications have been noted to adversely affect sperm health and function. Multiple classes of antibiotic medications have been shown to have potential for reversible decrease in sperm parameters. In cases of recurrent urinary tract infection, patients are prone to exposures to antibiotics and its attendant toxicities some of which affect testicular function. For example, nitrofurantoin is known to have gonadotoxic effect on the testes causing decrease sperm count and motility; similarly antibiotics like erythromycin, tetracycline, and the aminoglycosides disrupt sperm production with reduction in count and motility, while sulfa drugs decrease sperm count and motility and affect morphology. Also, prostate medications such as α-blockers have been shown to decrease the quality of semen parameters including sperm counts and motility. Similarly, the 5-α-reductase inhibitors like finasteride have been shown to decrease sperm quality even in low doses [35].

These factors in patients with BPH may collectively impair sperm production and functionality resulting in male infertility.

3.2 Relationship between BPH and erectile dysfunction

Erectile dysfunction (ED) and LUTS are conditions associated with significant negative impact on quality of life of patients and are known to have an increased prevalence in ageing men [33]. Although most drugs used in the treatment of BPH-associated LUTS have some negative impacts on patients' sexual function, studies have shown a strong causal relationship between LUTS due to BPH and sexual dysfunction. However, it is not clear how they are associated although there are emerging data supporting common pathophysiological mechanisms [36].

LUTS often coexist with ED in men with BPH and can themselves be an independent risk factor for erectile dysfunction. The prevalence and severity of both conditions increase with age, and with the severity of one condition often being associated with that of the other. Furthermore, when men seek treatment for one condition, they are often found to have both [37, 38].

Sexuality is an essential aspect of human relationships and has a significant impact on satisfaction. Men with moderate to severe LUTS are at increased risk for sexual dysfunction, including moderate to severe ED, ejaculatory dysfunction, and hypoactive sexual desire. Recent large-scale studies have shown a consistent and strong relationship between LUTS and both erectile dysfunction and ejaculatory dysfunction. It seems that the pathophysiological mechanisms of LUTS and BPH as well as certain treatments for these conditions may have an impact on both the erection and the ejaculatory component of the sexual response [39].

The pathophysiologic link between these conditions is not yet clear, but several theories have been described with various degrees of supporting data. There seems to be an overlap between the roles of these individual mechanisms, and the ultimate effect that leads to smooth muscle relaxation in prostatic, bladder neck, or erectile tissues. Mechanisms that have been proposed include the pelvic atherosclerosis theory and pelvic ischaemia, autonomic hyperactivity theory, calcium-independent Rho-kinase activation pathway, age-related hormone imbalances, and lastly, reduced nitric oxide (NO) levels [38].

The most explored of these mechanisms is the reduced nitric oxide levels. Nitric oxide is a noradrenergic, noncholinergic (NANC) mediator of smooth muscle activity and is present in the prostate, which also has nitric oxide synthetase activity. It is believed that prostatic smooth muscle tension is mediated by nitric oxide. Nitric oxide activates soluble guanylate cyclase (sGC) of smooth muscle cells, which in turn increases cyclic guanosine monophosphate (cGMP) levels ultimately resulting in smooth muscle cell relaxation, and this relaxation causes carvenous dilatation with consequent inflow of much blood and penile erection [40].

Additionally, PDE5-inhibitors were found in vitro to inhibit prostate stromal cell proliferation through attenuating and reverting fibroblast-to-myofibroblast trans-differentiation. The abundance of PDE5 iso-enzymes in the lower urinary tract and the inhibition of PDE5 in these tissues, leading to increased cGMP, have been demonstrated to reduce smooth muscle cell proliferation in the prostate; relax smooth muscle cells in the prostate, bladder neck, and supporting vasculature; and increase tissue oxygenation via improved blood perfusion and modulate bladder afferent nerve activity. The improvement of symptoms in patients with LUTS due to BPH treated with tadalafil is believed to be mediated by a combination of these effects [41, 42]. Moreover, they exert potent anti-inflammatory effects on the prostate thereby reducing fibrosis and overgrowth. All these beneficial effects help in maintaining prostatic structural anatomy and physiological activity [43].

3.3 Role of BPH in obstructive infertility

As the prostate enlarges, it compresses the urethra causing obstruction of not only urine but seminal fluid as well, or at least altering the direction of semen flow back into the bladder, and this can potentially cause male factor infertility as there is hindrance to the effective deposition of semen deep into the vagina during sexual intercourse.

In a few reports, there have been cases of recurrent urethritis in patients with benign prostatic hyperplasia developing ejaculatory duct obstruction by virtue of the inflammation that occurs at the level of the verumontanum where the openings of the ejaculatory ducts into the prostatic utricle are located.

Also, a common treatment for benign prostatic hyperplasia is transurethral resection of the prostate and although the therapeutic effect of this surgical method has been proven, it is traumatic, and cases of ejaculatory duct obstruction post TURP have been reported.

The obstruction of the ejaculatory ducts may result in azoospermia as in cases of bilateral obstruction or reduced seminal fluid volume (typically <2 ml) in solitary or incomplete obstruction with some spermatozoa present in the ejaculate. These situations can result in male factor infertility even though they are comparatively rare.

3.4 Impact of BPH-related treatments on ejaculation and male infertility

The most important sexual adverse effects of medical therapies are ejaculatory disorders after the use of some α-blockers and sexual desire impairment, erectile dysfunction, and ejaculatory disorders after the use of α-reductase inhibitors [44]. Several types of problems may occur with ejaculation: ejaculatory duct obstruction, retrograde ejaculation, retarded ejaculation, anejaculation, congenital anorgasmia, and painful ejaculation.

Most of the treatment options for LUTS due to BPH, both pharmacologic and surgical, are known to have significant sexual side effects and most importantly ejaculatory dysfunction. While ejaculatory dysfunction due to pharmacologic therapy is usually reversible on cessation of treatment, that attributable to surgical interventions is often permanent and irreversible [45]. The resultant effects of ejaculatory dysfunction are psychological stress and male infertility as the sperm is hindered from travelling out of the urethra into the vagina for possible fertilisation. The implicated treatments include the following.

3.4.1 Alpha-blockers

These are medications used for the treatment of BPH as well as hypertension. Alpha-blockers treat BPH by relaxing the prostatic capsule and bladder neck, thereby enlarging the channel through which the urine flows. However, when the bladder neck is relaxed, retrograde ejaculation can result. They can also decrease emission of sperm (transport of sperm from the vas deferens into the ejaculatory ducts), which can result in complete azoospermia without retrograde ejaculation. Most notorious of the group for this adverse effect are the selective blockers such as silodosin and tamsulosin. In some cases, they may cause complete anejaculation (no antegrade or retrograde flow of ejaculate with orgasm). Rates of ejaculatory dysfunction following use of tamsulosin and silodosin have generally been found to be about 10–30%. Ejaculatory dysfunction caused by alpha-blockers is typically reversed following stoppage of the medications.

3.4.2 5-alpha reductase inhibitors

The drugs notably finasteride and dutasteride are principally used in the treatment of LUTS due to BPH, commonly as a combination therapy. These drugs have the negative effects of erectile dysfunction, hypo-active sexual desire, and ejaculatory dysfunction including reduced, absent, or painful ejaculation, and these negatively impact on fertility [46].

3.4.3 Conventional surgical therapy

Even before any treatment consideration, LUTS due to BPH carries a risk of sexual dysfunction [47]. Most of the surgical interventions used in BPH management as long as they open the urinary channel can also damage the bladder neck further worsening the occurrences of sexual dysfunction. Such surgical treatments include transurethral resection of the prostate (TURP), laser prostate surgery such as HoLEP, microwave treatment of the prostate, transurethral needle ablation of the prostate (TUNA), and transurethral incision of the prostate (TUIP).

TURP has remained the gold standard treatment for BPH with regard to efficacy and safety [48]. Due to the fact that the ejaculatory ducts also empty into the prostatic urethra on either side of the verumontanum, ablation and excessive heat applied to the ejaculatory ducts may lead to charring, scarring, and duct obstruction with resultant anejaculation. Also, the bladder neck is known to physiologically close during ejaculation to propel the ejaculate forward to ensure deposition deep into the vagina. Unfortunately, during a TURP, resection of the bladder neck is commonly performed to further increase the calibre of the outflow tract and this leads to an incompetent bladder neck and resultant retrograde ejaculation. It has been shown that ejaculatory dysfunction occurs in up to 65% of post TURP patients of which about 50% do have retrograde ejaculation [45].

Holmium laser enucleation of the prostate (HoLEP), which is an alternative to TURP as it can be used for bigger sized prostate and for those at higher risk of bleeding, has been shown to have similar risks of ejaculatory dysfunction as TURP.

While transurethral incision of the prostate (TUIP) may be an option for symptomatic men with smaller prostate glands considering the bladder neck is incised and not resected, it is still associated with about 35% risk of ejaculatory dysfunction and can lead to irreversible ejaculatory dysfunction.

Open simple prostatectomy, which is still a viable option in some quarters especially in patients with very large glands or coexisting bladder pathology like diverticulum, is known to have an invariable high rate of ejaculatory dysfunction.

4. Diagnostic approach for male infertility due to BPH

4.1 Medical history and physical examination

The patient's detailed medical history should assess for symptoms of BPH, duration of infertility, and previous treatments, and rule out any risk factors and behavioural patterns that may impact his infertility. These factors include his lifestyle, family history (e.g. testicular cancer), comorbidities (e.g. hypertension, diabetes mellitus (DM), obesity, metabolic syndrome, testicular cancer, etc), genito-urinary infections (e.g. sexually transmitted infections), and history of testicular surgery, and exclude any potential known gonadotoxic medications or recreational drugs [49].

A focused urologic examination is mandatory in the assessment of every man with infertility due to BPH. The examination is aimed at eliciting findings suggestive of BPH, such as an enlarged prostate with benign features, and also ruling out other causes of infertility. Findings suggestive of other causes of infertility may include abnormal secondary sexual characteristics, abnormal testicular volume and/or consistency, testicular masses (suggestive of cancer), nodular, hard prostate (suggestive of cancer) absence of testes, gynaecomastia, varicocoele, etc.

4.2 Laboratory tests for hormonal evaluation

Hormonal evaluation should be performed for all male patients with infertility, whether due to BPH or not. The role of hormones in the pathogenesis of BPH has been well outlined. The imbalances in androgens, oestrogens, and gonadotrophins can affect spermatogenesis by various mechanisms. The level of serum testosterone, DHT, oestradiol, follicle-stimulating hormone(FSH), luteinizing hormone(LH) and prolactin should be checked. Thyroid function test can also be performed.

4.3 Semen analysis and evaluation of sperm parameters

The 6th edition of the WHO Manual for the Examination and Processing of Human Semen published in July 2021 is the working tool currently accepted

Parameter	2021 lower reference limit (95% CI)
Semen volume (mL)	1.4 (1.3–1.5)
Total sperm number (10^6/mL)	39 (35–40)
Sperm concentration (10^6/mL)	16 (15–18)
Total motility (PR + NP, %)	42 (40–43)
Progressive motility (PR. %)	30 (29–31)
Vitality (live spermatozoa, %)	54 (50–56)
Sperm morphology (normal forms, %)	4 (3.9–4.0)

NP, non-progressive; PR, progressive.

Table 1.
Lower reference limits (5th centiles and their 95% CIs) for semen characteristics.

worldwide for the analysis of semen. Semen analysis remains the cornerstone of male infertility evaluation. The basic examination would assess for semen volume, sperm numbers, sperm motility, sperm morphology, and sperm vitality. The normal reference ranges are as shown in **Table 1** [50].

One test is adequate if the semen analysis meets WHO criteria. If at least two test findings are abnormal, further andrological evaluation would be indicated. It is worthy to be noted that no single sperm parameter, such as concentration, morphology, or motility, can be used to diagnose infertility in and on itself.

Advanced evaluation of sperm parameters includes measurement of sperm DNA fragmentation index, assessment of reactive oxygen species (ROS), membrane ion channels, acrosome reaction and sperm chromatin structure and stability, and computer-assisted sperm analysis (CASA). Genetic analysis may be indicated depending on the clinical findings and semen parameters [51].

4.4 Imaging techniques to assess BPH and its impact on fertility

Imaging modalities may help to assess the severity and extent of BPH and its impact on fertility. The main role of imaging is the identification of the causes of infertility.

Transrectal ultrasound scan (TRUS) can be used to evaluate the prostate gland (prostate volume, nodularity, cysts, etc.) and its adjoining structures. It can also be used in patients with low seminal volume, acidic PH, and severe oligo-zoospermia or azoospermia, in whom obstruction is suspected. Patients with congenital bilateral absence of vas deferens (CBAVD), abnormalities of the epididymis, seminal vesicles can also be assessed via TRUS.

Scrotal ultrasound scan is the most commonly performed imaging modality where causes of infertility other than BPH are suspected. It is employed to assess for testicular volume and testicular/scrotal masses like cancer, cysts, varicocoele, as well as assessment of obstructive azoospermia [51].

MR imaging of the brain is very beneficial for evaluating pertinent neurologic abnormalities, such as pituitary gland disorders, that are suspected on the basis of hormone analysis results [52].

5. Management of male infertility due to BPH and BPH-related treatments

5.1 Medical management of BPH to improve fertility

Male infertility due to BPH can be treated when the underlying pathology being BPH is addressed. As outlined earlier the medical therapy of BPH includes the use of α1-adrenoceptor blockers, which relax prostatic smooth muscles e.g. tamsulosin alone, or in combination with 5α-reductase inhibitors, which reduce prostate volume, e.g. finasteride. Others such as muscarinic receptor antagonists e.g. oxybutynin, β-3 agonists e.g. mirabegon, phosphodiesterase 5 inhibitors e.g. tadalafil, and some plant extracts e.g. saw palmetto [32] may play roles in improving symptoms.

Anti-androgens and aromatase inhibitors can also be used.

It is worthy of note to mention here that the treatment of some co-morbid conditions like metabolic syndrome (metS) associated with BPH have been found to improve infertility in these patients. Lifestyle modifications like smoking cessation, weight loss and the use of medications such as anti-hypertensives, euglycaemic agents and lipid lowering drugs have excellent results in the improvement of semen parameters [53].

5.2 Use of medications to enhance semen count and quality

Over the years, some medications have been shown to directly or indirectly improve sperm parameters such as sperm count and concentration, motility, as well as morphology. These agents can be broadly placed into 2 groups: hormone mediated agents and antioxidant based supplements.

5.2.1 Hormone mediated agents

These medications help to improve sperm count or quality and they include the selective oestrogen receptor modulators like clomiphene citrate, FSH, selective aromatase inhibitors such as anastrozole and HCG.

Clomiphene citrate is used by most urologists even as an off label medication to treat male infertility. It blocks oestrogen from interacting with the pituitary gland and consequently increases testosterone, luteinizing hormone(LH) and follicular stimulating hormone(FSH) levels. It has been shown to improve sperm concentration and motility by 4–5%. This boost can be of utmost value in oligospermic patients or those with poor motility towards achieving pregnancy. It may also help azoospermia patients resume sperm production thus improving the chances for successful sperm extraction [54].

FSH is known to help in stimulating testicular growth even though minimally and aid sperm production and thereby improve pregnancy outcomes in patients with hypogonadism, oligospermia, and oligoasthenoteratospermia.

Similarly, anastrozole and letrozole are known to decrease oestrogen production and increase testosterone production. They have been found to help correct hormonal imbalances and improve sperm concentration in sub-fertile men [55].

Human chorionic gonadotropin (HCG) is known to improve testosterone levels in men with secondary hypogonadism without the adverse effect of suppression of the hypothalamic-pituitary-gonadal axis as seen with exogenous testosterone therapy while also improving sperm production.

5.2.2 Antioxidant based supplements

Oxidative stress is known to occur following the production of reactive oxygen species (ROS) which exceeds the body's natural antioxidant defences. ROS are produced from environmental factors such as high temperature, electromagnetic waves, air pollution, insecticides, alcohol consumption, obesity, as well as poor nutrition, and these impact negatively on testicular function with resultant increase in sperm DNA fragmentation, abnormal sperm morphological forms, and decrease in sperm concentration and motility with an overall negative impact on male fertility.

There are natural antioxidants in semen and these include vitamin E, vitamin C, superoxide dismutase, glutathione and thioredoxin. These antioxidants play critical roles in neutralising the activities of free radicals and protect sperm from ROS that are already produced [56].

Recently, attention has been drawn to the effect of oxidative stress on male infertility and the role played by the use of oral antioxidant supplements in the improvement of semen parameters in infertile men, and most of these studies have shown a positive relationship between antioxidants and improved male fertility outcomes [57].

Antioxidants in supplements have become a common prescription by urologists to males who are being managed for infertility in a bid to improve testicular function and sperm parameters. Notable components of these supplements are vitamin C, vitamin E, L- carnitine, Coenzyme Q10, zinc, selenium and N-acetyl-cysteine. Others include lycopene, vitamin D, D- aspartic acid and folate.

There are numerous studies to support the positive impact of use of these supplements in improving semen parameters and pregnancy outcomes in infertile males. A study conducted in 2006 showed that use of 1000 mg twice daily vitamin C for 2 months caused sperm count to double with an increase in motility of 90%. Its combination with vitamin E has been shown to be very effective in reducing sperm DNA fragmentation. Similarly, studies have shown that vitamin E combined with selenium results in total improvement of sperm motility and morphology and causes a 10.8% increase in spontaneous pregnancy rate when compared to a non-treatment group.

In a study done by Balercia and colleagues on the effect of CoQ10 on sperm motility in infertile men, 60 men with asthenoteratospermia reviewed showed an improvement in the semen concentration and sperm motility with the occurrence of 12 spontaneous pregnancies [58]. Lycopene has been shown to decrease oxidative stress and sperm DNA damage, and cause an increase in sperm count, concentration, motility and morphology, while vitamin D has been shown to improve motility in men with asthenospermia.

Folate helps sperm production and improves sperm concentrations in infertile males. Zinc is known to help immune function, and its use is associated with significant improvements in semen volume, sperm motility and sperm morphology.

5.3 Surgical interventions to alleviate BPH-related infertility

The surgery of BPH can be employed in treating infertility in the surgically amendable cases. These surgeries include resection, enucleation, vaporisation, alternative ablative techniques, and non-ablative techniques [32]. Transurethral resection of the prostate (TURP) is the gold standard method for surgically treating BPH. These surgeries would reduce the size of the prostate, reduce the burden of inflammation, and thus improve the fertility profile of the patient. Some complications of these surgeries can also lead to situations that would cause infertility.

Such complications include retrograde ejaculation, ejaculatory duct stricture, urethral stricture, etc. There is paucity of data regarding the achievable pregnancy rates following surgical interventions in infertility caused by BPH. This serves as grounds for further research.

Bariatric surgeries may be indicated in patients with metS and have been noted to improve infertility in this group of patients [59].

5.4 Assisted reproductive technology for couples affected by BPH-related infertility

Assisted reproductive technology (ART) are a set of protocols or procedures that involve the in vitro handling or manipulation of human oocytes, sperm, or embryos, with the intent of establishing pregnancy. This is indicated in situations where the above options of treatment fail. Various techniques of ART exist and they include intrauterine insemination (IUI), in vitro fertilisation (IVF), intracytoplasmic sperm injection (ICSI), testicular sperm extraction (TESE), and percutaneous epididymal sperm aspiration (PESA).

6. Measures, therapies, and mitigating interventions for BPH treatment related infertility

Over the years, various measures have been identified that can be put into place to either prevent or mitigate the occurrence and negative impact on fertility among male patients treated for benign prostatic hyperplasia.

6.1 Treatment of retrograde ejaculation

6.1.1 Discontinue alpha-blocker medications

Terazosin, doxazosin, and alfuzosin are known to have lower rates of ejaculatory dysfunction when compared to other alpha-blockers, and this has been attributed to the non-specific mechanism of action of the medications. The more selective and the higher the affinity of the drug to the alpha 1a receptors, the greater the likelihood of ejaculatory dysfunction.

Tamsulosin and silodosin are the alpha-blockers most likely to result in ejaculatory problems. In cases of mild to moderate symptoms, the alpha-blocker can be temporarily stopped until pregnancy is achieved, and this usually is the most effective approach. In men with more severe urinary voiding problems, switching to a less selective alpha-blocker, such as alfuzosin, can often help resolve the ejaculatory problems [60].

6.1.2 Use of alpha agonists

Alpha agonists work by increasing the strength of bladder neck closure during ejaculation. The success rate in reversing retrograde ejaculation is about 20–30%. Intermittent short courses of treatment are recommended to maximise benefit. Examples of alpha agonists include pseudoephedrine, phenylpropanolamine, ephedrine sulphate, and imipramine. Of these agents, the most commonly used is pseudoephedrine and it is given for 2–7 days' duration. The drug can be used prior to semen analysis (to assess treatment response), in conjunction with timed intercourse [60].

6.1.3 Urine sperm retrieval and assisted reproductive techniques

Sperm can be collected at the time of a semen analysis and then used with intrauterine insemination. The urine must however first be alkalinized prior to specimen collection, as urine is acidic, and this acidity is damaging to sperm. Common agents for urine alkalinization are oral baking soda and sodium bicarbonate tablets or capsules. They are typically taken the night before and 1–2 hours before ejaculation.

6.2 Treatment of ejaculatory duct obstruction

Several different treatment options are available, including ejaculatory duct dilation, transurethral resection of the ejaculatory duct (TURED), and sperm extraction combined with IVF/ICSI [61].

6.2.1 Ejaculatory duct dilation

This entails passing long, thin probes into the ejaculatory ducts under cystoscopic guidance and progressively passing larger probes in an attempt to dilate any narrowing of the ejaculatory ducts. Recent modifications include use of small inflatable balloons.

6.2.2 Sperm extraction and IVF

Men with ejaculatory duct obstruction typically have normal sperm production. One option is to bypass the obstruction and proceed with sperm extraction combined with IVF/ICSI. This approach avoids the need for TURED with its possible complications.

6.2.3 Transurethral resection of the ejaculatory duct (TURED)

This is done usually on an outpatient basis under anaesthesia and involves the use of a resectoscope with careful resection of portions of the ejaculatory ducts using electrocautery or a laser, thereby relieving the blockage. This procedure is often combined with the injection of coloured dye into the seminal vesicles by TRUS prior to the resection. Therefore, when the obstruction has been successfully removed, this coloured dye can be seen through the scope flowing through the newly opened ejaculatory ducts.

6.3 Novel therapies for BPH management

6.3.1 Prostatic urethral lift (Urolift)

This is a newer BPH treatment characterized by the use of non-thermal method to cystoscopically lay implant trans-prostatic suture to widen the prostatic lumen by compressing the prostatic tissue in a bid to mechanically open the prostate. Though the data are preliminary, sexual and ejaculatory side effects are reported to be minimal [61, 62].

6.3.2 Water vapour thermal energy treatment (Rezum)

It is typically used for prostates less than 80 g. It involves the use of radiofrequency generated thermal energy delivered transurethrally to ablate the prostate. Sexual function is preserved because the thermal effects are not transmitted beyond the targeted areas. In the majority of men, sexual and ejaculatory functions are preserved [AUA Update 2019] [63].

6.3.3 Aquablation

This is a recently developed system that utilizes high pressure water jet technology to precisely cut and resect prostate tissue. Since thermal energy is not used, the sexual adverse effects are therefore minimized. Studies in this regard are still few and evidence at the moment are limited [64, 65].

6.3.4 Urethral-sparing simple prostatectomy

This is performed via a minimally invasive robotic approach, in which the seminal vesicles, urethra, and ejaculatory ducts are preserved. It should be noted that studies are limited and that ejaculatory outcomes are heavily dependent on the surgeon's technique and expertise as well as prostatic anatomy [66].

6.3.5 Hood-sparing technique

This technique may be employed for both TURP and HoLEP. Avoiding damage to the paracollicular and supracollicular tissue proximal to the verumontanum (ejaculatory hood), it is believed to preserve antegrade ejaculation. Although a hood sparing approach with these interventions seems to be promising, results are mixed and require ongoing further investigation [67].

7. Conclusion

Benign prostatic hyperplasia (BPH) indeed has a negative impact on male fertility. Prostatic enlargement can potentially hinder the transport of sperm during ejaculation, affecting the chances of successful conception. Additionally, medications used in its management and management of its associated complications may affect sperm quality or motility, further complicating fertility issues. Sadly, known standard surgical interventions for BPH are major potentiators to male infertility leaving the individual patients and urologists with limited options towards ameliorating this burden. Consequently, it becomes imperative to fully understand the enormity of the challenge, mechanisms by which they occur, as well as available management options with a view to maximising available options towards improved outcomes and patient satisfaction.

An intact sexual function, especially ejaculation, is critical in the domain of male fertility. Impediments to semen outflow, whether it is ejaculatory dysfunction or erectile dysfunction, will cause significant challenges for men attempting to conceive. There are multiple organic sources of such dysfunction, but it is important to identify the iatrogenic causes as well, such as lower urinary tract symptoms due to BPH and its treatments.

While the alpha-blockers carry a significant risk of ejaculatory dysfunction, the non-selective agents appear to have less of such negative effect. With regard to surgical therapeutic options, there is strong evidence to show that Turps and HoLEPs can lead to ejaculatory dysfunction and that alternative treatments such as prostatic urethral lift, water vapour therapy, and aquablation may provide adequate treatment for patients with LUTS attributable to BPH while preserving ejaculatory function and by extension male fertility. This evidence is strongest for prostatic urethral lift, followed by water vapour treatment, while aquablation requires further research.

Conflict of interest

The authors declare no conflict of interest.

Author details

Julius Akhaine[1*] and Ifiok Umana[2]

1 Division of Urology, Department of Surgery, Federal Medical Centre, Keffi, Nasarawa State, Nigeria

2 Division of Urology, Department of Surgery, Jos University Teaching Hospital, Jos, Plateau State, Nigeria

*Address all correspondence to: akhasj2017@gmail.com

IntechOpen

© 2024 The Author(s). Licensee IntechOpen. This chapter is distributed under the terms of the Creative Commons Attribution License (http://creativecommons.org/licenses/by/4.0), which permits unrestricted use, distribution, and reproduction in any medium, provided the original work is properly cited.

References

[1] Yeboah E. The prostate gland. In: Archeampong EQ, Naaeder SA, Ugwu BT, editors. Principles and Practice of Surgery Including Pathology in the Tropics. 5th ed. Accra: Ghana Publishing Cooperative; 2015. pp. 969-997

[2] Ferré-Dolcet L, Frigotto L, Contiero B, Bedin S, Romagnoli S. Prostatic fluid composition and semen quality in dogs with benign prostatic hyperplasia undergoing treatment with osaterone acetate. Reproduction in Domestic Animals. 2021;**57**(1):72-79

[3] Roehrborn CG, Strand DW. Benign prostatic hyperplasia: Etiology, pathophysiology, epidemiology, and natural history. In: Partin AW, Dmochowski RR, Kavoussi LR, Peters CA, editors. Campbell-Wash-Wein Urology. 12th ed. Philadelphia: Elsevier; 2021. p. 5084

[4] Manley JP, Rowe EW, Bachi CA. Anatomy of the prostate. In: Keane TE, Graham SD, editors. Glenn's Urological Surgery. 8th ed. Philadelphia: Wolters Kluwers; 2016. pp. 435-442

[5] Ashley ER, Ronald R. Development, molecular biology, and physiology of the prostate. In: Wein AJ, Kavoussi LR, Partin AW, editors. Campbell-Walsh Urology. 11th ed. Philadephia: Elsevier; 2016. pp. 2393-2324

[6] Patel ND, Parsons JK. Epidemiology and etiology of benign prostatic hyperplasia and bladder outlet obstruction. Indian Journal of Urology. 2014;**30**(2):170-176. DOI: 10.4103/0970-1591.126900

[7] Lee SWH, Chan EMC, Lai YK. The global burden of lower urinary tract symptoms suggestive of benign prostatic hyperplasia: A systematic review and meta-analysis. Scientific Reports. 2017;**7**(1):7984. DOI: 10.1038/s41598-017-06628-8

[8] Awedew AF, Han H, Abbasi B, Abbasi-Kangevari M, Ahmed MB, Almidani O, et al. The global, regional, and national burden of benign prostatic hyperplasia in 204 countries and territories from 2000 to 20219: A systematic analysis for the global burden of disease study 2019. The Lancet Healthy Longevity. 2022;**3**(11):e754-e776

[9] World Health Organization. International Classification of Diseases and Related Health Problems, 11th Revision (ICD-11). Geneva, Switzerland: World Health Organization; 2019

[10] World Health Organisation. WHO Laboratory Manual for the Examination of Human Semen and Sperm-Cervical Interaction. United Kingdom: Cambridge University Press; 1999

[11] Hata J, Harigane Y, Matsuoka K, Akaihata H, Yaginuma K, Meguro S, et al. Mechanism of androgen-independent stromal proliferations in benign prostatic hyperplasia. International Journal of Molecular Sciences. 2023;**24**:11634

[12] Horton R, Hsieh P, Barberia J, Pages L, Cosgrove M. Altered blood androgens in elderly men with prostate hyperplasia. The Journal of Clinical Endocrinology and Metabolism. 1975;**41**:793-796

[13] Hammond GL, Kontturi M, Vihko P, Vihko R. Serum steroids in normal males and patients with prostatic diseases. Clinical Endocrinology. 1978;**9**:113-121

[14] Robert RO, Jacobson DJ, Rhodes T, Klee GG, Leiber MM, Jacobsen SJ. Serum

sex hormones and measures of benign prostatic hyperplasia. The Prostate. 2004;**61**:124-131

[15] King KJ, Nicholson HD, Assinder SJ. Effect of increasing ratio of estrogen: Androgen on proliferation of normal human prostate stromal and epithelial cells, and the malignant cell line LNCaP. Prostate. 2006;**66**:105-114

[16] Rastrelli G, Vignozzi L, Corona G, Maggi M. Testosterone and benign prostatic hyperplasia. Sexual Medicine Reviews. 2019;7:259-271

[17] Kumar S, Yadav RN, Gupta P, Gasper BL, Kakkar N, Verma A, et al. Prostatic hyperplasia in acromegaly, a myth or reality: A case-control study. European Journal of Endocrinology. 2015;**172**:97-106

[18] Ropiquet F, Giri D, Lamb DJ, Ittmann M. FGF7 and FGF2 are increased in benign prostatic hyperplasia and are associated with increased proliferation. The Journal of Urology. 1990;**162**:595-599

[19] Kim SK, Park HK, Choi HS, Yoo KH, Chung JH. Association study of polymorphism of epidermal growth factor and epidermal growth factor receptor with benign prostatic hyperplasia in a Korean population. International Neurourology Journal. 2016;**20**:363-370

[20] De Nunzio C, Presicce F, Tubaro A. Inflammatory mediators in the development and progression of benign prostatic hyperplasia. Nature Reviews. Urology. 2016;**13**:613-626

[21] Kohnen PW, Drach GW. Patterns of inflammation in prostate hyperplasia: A histologic and bacteriologic study. The Journal of Urology. 1979;**121**:755-760

[22] Nickel JC, Roehrborn CG, O'Leary MP, Bostwick DG, Somerville MC, Rittmaster RS. The relationship between prostate inflammation and lower urinary tract symptoms: Examination of baseline data from the REDUCE trial. European Urology. 2008;**54**:1379-1384

[23] Torkko KC, Wilson RS, Smith EE, Kusek JW, van Bokhoven A, Lucia MS. Prostate biopsy markers of inflammation are associated with risk of clinical progression of benign prostatic hyperplasia: Findings from the MTOPS study. The Journal of Urology. 2015;**194**:454-461

[24] Penna G, Fibbi B, Amuchastegui S, Cossetti C, Aquilano F, Laverny G, et al. Human benign prostatic hyperplasia stromal cells as inducers and targets of chronic immune-mediated inflammation. Journal of Immunology. 2009;**182**:4056-4064

[25] Fowke JH, Murff HJ, Signorello LB, Lund L, Blot WJ. Race and socioeconomic status are independently associated with benign prostatic hyperplasia. The Journal of Urology. 2008;**180**:2091-2096

[26] Hellwege JN, Stallings S, Torstenson ES, Carroll R, Borthwick KM, Brilliant MH, et al. Heritability and genome-wide association study of benign prostatic hyperplasia (BPH) in the eMERGE network. Scientific Reports. 2019;**9**:6077

[27] Takezaka K, Fujita K, Matushita M, Motooka D, Hatano K, Banno E, et al. The firmicutes/bacteroides ration of the human gut microbiota is associated with prostate enlargement. The Prostate. 2021;**81**:1267-1293

[28] Tsai KY, Wu DC, Wu WJ, Wang JW, Juan YS, Li CC, et al. Exploring the association between gut and urine microbiota and prostatic disease

including benign prostatic hyperplasia and prostate cancer using 16S rRNA sequencing. Biomedicine. 2022;**10**:2676

[29] Okada K, Takeawa K, Tsujimura G, Imanaka T, Kuribayashi S, Ueda N, et al. Localisation and potential role of prostate microbiota. Frontiers in Cellular and Infection Microbiology. 2022;**12**:1048319

[30] Jain S, Samal AG, Das B, Pradhan B, Sahu N, Mohapatra D, et al. *Escherichia coli*, a common constituent of benign prostatic hyperplasia-associated microbiota induces inflammation and DNA damage in prostate epithelialc ells. The Prostate. 2020;**80**:1341-1352

[31] Yao MW, Green JSA. How international is the international prostate symptom score? A literature review of validated translations of the IPSS, the most widely used self-administered patient questionnaire for male lower urinary tract symptoms. LUTS: Lower Urinary Tract Symptoms. 2022;**14**(2):92-101

[32] Cornu JN, Gacci M, Hashim H, Hermann TRW, Malde S, Netsch C, et al. Non-neurogenic Male Lower Urinary Tract Symptoms (LUTS). EAU Guidelines. ISBN 978-94-92671-23-3. Arnhem, The Netherlands: EAU Guidelines Office; CAP3, 2024:5-124. Available from: https://uroweb.org/guidelines

[33] Hoover P, Naz RK. Do men with prostate abnormalities (prostatitis/benign prostatic hyperplasia/prostate cancer) develop immunity to spermatozoa or seminal plasma? International Journal of Andrology. 2012;**35**:608-615. ISSN 0105-6263. DOI: 10.1111/j.1365-2605.2011.01246.x

[34] Ruben DM, Florencia CS, Maria LB, Juan PM. Implications of prostate inflammation on male fertility. Andrologia. 2018;**50**(11):e13093. DOI: 10.1111/and.1309

[35] Jiayi D, Xuejun S, Zhanhu Z, Hua J, Jun S. FDA-approved medications that impair human spermatogenesis. 2017;**8**(6):10714-10725. DOI: 10.18632/oncotarget.12956

[36] Claus G, Overborne M. Benign prostatic hyperplasia: Etiology, pathophysiology, epidemiology, and natural history. In: Wein AJ, Kavoussi LR, Partin AW, editors. Campbell-Walsh Urology. 11th ed. Elsevier; 2016. pp. 2425-2462

[37] Hatzimouratidis K. A review of the use of tadalafil in the treatment of benign prostatic hyperplasia in men with and without erectile dysfunction. Therapeutic Advances in Urology. 2014;**6**:135-147

[38] Hofner K, Claes H, De Reijke TM, Folkestad B, Speakman MJ. Tamsulosin 0.4 mg once daily: Effect on sexual function in patients with lower urinary tract symptoms suggestive of benign prostatic obstruction. European Urology. 1999;**36**(4):335-341

[39] Lee SW, Paick JS, Park HJ, Won JE, Morisaki Y, Sorsaburu S, et al. The efficacy and safety of Tadalafil 5 mg once daily in Korean men with lower urinary tract symptoms suggestive of benign prostatic hyperplasia: An integrated analysis. World Journal of Mens Health. 2014;**32**(1):28

[40] McNicholas T, Speakman MJ, Kirby RS. Evaluation and nonsurgical management of benign prostatic hyperplasia. In: Wein AJ, Kavoussi LR, Partin AW, editors. Campbell-Walsh Urology. 11th ed. Philadelphia: Elsevier; 2016. pp. 2463-2503

[41] Wang H, Chang Y, Liang H. Tamsulosin and solifenacin in the

treatment of benign prostatic hyperplasia in combination with overactive bladder. Pakistan Journal of Medical Science. 2017;**33**(4):988-992

[42] Rosen RC, Giuliano F, Carson CC. Sexual dysfunction and lower urinary tract symptoms (LUTS) associated with benign prostatic hyperplasia (BPH). European Urology. 2005;**47**:824-837

[43] Yokoyama O, Igawa Y, Takeda M, Yamaguchi T, Murakami M, Viktrup L. Tadalafil for lower urinary tract symptoms secondary to benign prostatic hyperplasia: A review of clinical data in Asian men and an update on the mechanism of action. Therapeutic Advances in Urology. 2015;**7**:249-264

[44] Mauro G, Ian E, Francois G, Dimitris H, Steven A. Critical analysis of the relationship between sexual dysfunctions and lower urinary tract symptoms due to benign prostatic hyperplasia. European Urology. 2011;**60**(4):809-825. DOI: 10.1016/j.euro.2011.06.037

[45] Priyanka B, Gabriella JA. The role of benign prostatic hyperplasia on ejaculatory dysfunction;**116**(3):611-617. DOI: 10.1016/j.fertnstert.2021.07.1199

[46] Corona G, Tirabassi G, Santi D, Maseroli E, Gacci M, Dicuio M, et al. Sexual dysfunction in subjects treated with inhibitors of 5α-reductase for benign prostatic hyperplasia: A comprehensive review and meta-analysis. Andrology. 2017;**5**:671-678

[47] Rosen RC, Fitzpatrick JM. Ejaculatory dysfunction in men with lower urinary tract symptoms suggestive of benign prostatic hyperplasia. BJU International. 2009;**104**:974-983

[48] Foster HE, Barry MJ, Dahm P, Gandhi MC, Kaplan SA, Kohler TS, et al. Surgical management of lower urinary tract symptoms attributed to benign prostatic hyperplasia: AUA guideline. The Journal of Urology. 2018;**200**:612-619

[49] Kasman AM, Zhang CA, Li S, Lu Y, Lathi RB, Stevenson DK, et al. Association between preconception paternal health and pregnancy loss in the USA: An analysis of US claims data. Human Reproduction. 2021;**36**(3):785. DOI: 10.1093/humrep/deaa332

[50] World Health Organisation. WHO Laboratory Manual for the Examination and Processing of Human Semen. 6th ed. Geneva: World Health Organisation; 2021. Available from: https://www.who.int/publications/i/item/97892400030787

[51] Salonia A, Bettocchi C, Capogrosso P, Carvalho J, Corona G, Dinkelman-Smith M, et al. Sexual and reproductive health. In: EAU Guidelines. ISBN 978-94-92671-23-3. Arnhem, The Netherlands: EAU Guidelines Office; 2024. Available from: https://uroweb.org/guidelines

[52] Mittal PK, Little B, Harri PA, Miller PA, Alexander LF, Kalb B, et al. Role of imaging in the evaluation of male infertility. Radiographics. 2017;**37**(3):837-854

[53] Service CA, Puri D, Al Azzawi S, Hsiesh T, Patel DP. The impact of obesity and metabolic health on male fertility: A systematic review. Fertility and Sterility. 2023;**120**(6):1098-1111

[54] Manou H, Roel LN, Huijsmans M, Tycho W, Lock T. Clomiphene citrate for male infertility: A systematic review and meta-analysis. Andrology. 2023. DOI: 10.1111/andr.13388

[55] Raman JD, Schlegel PN. Aromatase inhibitors for male infertility. Jurology.

2002;**167**:624-629. DOI: 10.1016/s0022-5347/02/1672-0624/0

[56] Tremellen K. Oxidative stress and male infertility-a clinical perspective. Human Reproduction Update. 2008;**14**:243-258

[57] Sedigheh A, Reihane B, Akram G. Antioxidant supplements and semen parameters: An evidence based review. International Journal of Reproductive Biomedicine. 2016;**14**(12):729-736

[58] Balercia G, Buldreghini E, Vignini A, Tiano L, Paggi F, Amoroso S, et al. Coenzyme Q 10 treatment in infertile men with idiopathic asthenozoospermia: A placebo-controlled, double-blind randomized trial. Fertility and Sterility. 2009;**91**:1785-1792

[59] Moxthe L, Sauls R, Ruiz M, Stern M, Gonzalvo J, et al. Effects of bariatric surgeries on male and female fertility: A systematic review. Journal of Reproduction & Infertility. 2020;**21**(2):71-86

[60] Amanda J, Dimitrios S, Peter W. The management of retrograde ejaculation: A systematic review and update. Fertility and Sterility. 2012;**97**:306-312.e6

[61] Overborne CG, Gange SN, Shore ND, Giddens JL, Bolton DM, Cowan BE, et al. The prostatic urethral lift for the treatment of lower urinary tract symptoms associated with prostate enlargement due to benign prostatic hyperplasia: The LIFT study. The Journal of Urology. 2013;**190**:2161-2216

[62] Roehrborn CG, Rukstalis DB, Barkin J, Gange SN, Shore ND, Giddens JL, et al. Three year results of the prostatic urethral LIFT study. The Canadian Journal of Urology. 2015;**22**:7772-7782

[63] McVary KT, Rogers T, Overborne CG. Rezūm water vapor thermal therapy for lower urinary tract symptoms associated with benign prostatic hyperplasia: 4-year results from randomized controlled study. Urology. 2019;**126**:171-179

[64] Gilling P, Barber N, Bidair M, Anderson P, Sutton M, Aho T, et al. WATER: A double-blind, randomized, controlled trial of aquablation ® vs transurethral resection of the prostate in benign prostatic hyperplasia. The Journal of Urology. 2018;**199**(5):1252-1261

[65] Hwang EC, Jung JH, Borofsky M, Kim MH, Dahm P. Aquablation of the prostate for the treatment of lower urinary tract symptoms in men with benign prostatic hyperplasia. Cochrane Database of Systematic Reviews. 2019:2CD013143

[66] Porpiglia F, Checcucci E, Amparore D, Niculescu G, Volpi G, Piramide F, et al. Urethral-sparing robot-assisted simple prostatectomy: An innovative technique to preserve ejaculatory function overcoming the limitation of the standard Millin approach. European Urology. 2021;**80**:222-233

[67] Kim M, Song SH, Ku JH, Kim HJ, Paick JS. Pilot study of the clinical efficacy of ejaculatory hood sparing technique for ejaculation preservation in holmium laser enucleation of the prostate. International Journal of Impotence Research. 2015;**27**:20-24

Section 3

New Strategies for Prostate Cancer

Chapter 7

Localized Prostate Cancer: A Clinically Significant Disease and Emerging Imaging Modalities

Sergio Contreras

Abstract

A trend has emerged toward the timely diagnosis of prostate cancer. Worldwide, early stages represent more than two-thirds of all prostate cancers. Novel software, highly sensitive images, or techniques available for its detection could lead to over-diagnosis of clinically irrelevant diseases. Conversely, inadequate staging could miss advanced diseases. Selecting a treatment for prostate cancer can be a difficult task, some prostate cancer may not require treatment, especially considering that treating early stages may not impact the patient's longevity. A multidisciplinary approach, supported by sophisticated imaging and diagnostic techniques and their correlation with biochemical, pathological, and clinical parameters, helps to define the risk. These risk groups are essential when selecting a definitive or radical treatment. These treatment modalities may include a combination of radiotherapy, hormonal therapies, surgery, or simply observation. For each of these options, the toxicity profile, side effects, quality of life, and survival must be considered. All these variables must be taken into account when defining treatment. Additionally, the intensification of treatment is a recent addition to the standard treatment of high-risk prostate cancer. Therefore, appropriate risk characterization is essential.

Keywords: high-risk, intermediate-risk, localized-prostate-cancer, radiotherapy plus ADT, mpMRI

1. Introduction

Worldwide, the age-standardized incidence rate of prostate cancer is 30.7 per 100,000 males [1]. According to data from the National Cancer Institute/ Surveillance, Epidemiology, and End Results (NCI/SEER, 2009–2015), up to 77% are localized with no evidence of lymph node involvement [2].

Clinically significant prostatic cancer involves those with stages higher than T2N0M0 with Gleason scores more advanced than 3 + 3 or ISUP 2 (international society of urological pathology group 2), and specific prostatic antigens with values over 10 ng/ml. The idea of treating clinically significant diseases lies in the probability of specific cancer death (SCD). Currently, we know that beyond 10 year of follow-up, SCD has been reported as 19.6% (95% CI, 18.0–21.2) for intermediate-risk disease and 35.5% (95% CI, 34.2.2–36.8) for high-risk disease [3]. Therefore, enhancing effective diagnostic tests for high-risk diseases to predict specific cancer deaths is justified.

2. Staging the disease

Evidence has previously been reported for the emerging multiparametric MRI (mpMRI), demonstrating its usefulness in active surveillance by diminishing unnecessary biopsies. The mpMRI diminished clinically insignificant prostate cancers by 9% and avoided 37% of biopsies in men. Efforts to decrease overtreatment and initiate timely treatment in localized diseases that are considered clinically significant should be the focus of curative treatment.

The burden of permanent complications should be considered in advance of definitive therapy. Ruling out metastatic disease is a mandatory element of the workup. Currently, the PET agents, 68Ga-PSMA-11 and 18F-DCFPyL, have been approved by the US Food and Drug Administration for newly diagnosed high-risk prostate cancers [4, 5]. The PROSTAGE trial reported sensibility for PSMA PET CT of 0.90 (0.78–1.00), with AUC values for bone metastasis detection of 0.90 (95% confidence interval [CI]: 0.85–0.95) [6].

Relevant data for lower-risk prostate cancer, such as the intermediate-risk group, was obtained from a retrospective study. Researchers studied diagnosed unfavorable intermediate-risk patients who underwent PSMA PET/CT as a primary staging modality to identify independent predictors of metastatic disease. In multivariable analysis, two variables were statistically significant: staging T3 with an OR of 2.72 [95% CI, 1.27–5.83] and >50% positive prostate biopsies with an OR of 3.87 [95% CI, 1.74–8.62]. Among all patients staged with PSMA PET, 9.3% had metastatic disease [7]. Therefore, the unfavorable risk group should undergo staging with this imaging technique.

3. Surgery or not

Analysis of data from the PREVENTER trial identifies that 20% of complications are associated with a prostatectomy procedure regardless of the type (robotic vs. opened). In multivariable logistic regression, the pathological stage T3b (OR 2.76, 95% CI 1.23–6.00; $P = 0.01$) was identified as a predictor of postoperative complications [8]. Therefore, which patients should avoid a surgical approach without detrimental effects on overall survival while preserving good quality of life?

This question should be approached by first conceiving a curative procedure, which means ensuring no evidence of residual disease, clear margins, and minimal risk of microscopic lymph node involvement. This curative approach considers preventing the need for additional radiotherapy and its subsequent toxicities when offered as an adjuvant or salvage treatment. Tools such as nomograms have been developed to select the best candidates for curative procedures and identify those at risk of poor outcomes. However, the limitations of nomograms are well-known.

Four validated nomograms have been compared for diagnostic accuracy. All nomograms (MSKCC and Briganti Nomograms from 2012, 2017, and 2019) showed high sensitivity ($Se > 0.90$) but low specificity ($Sp < 0.20$) and similar AUC (range: 0.526–0.573) in predicting pN+. Notably, the MSKCC prediction did not vary significantly between pN0 and pN+ groups ($p = 0.2$). These nomograms had low specificity in predicting lymph node involvement, which is why prostatic lymph node dissection is considered the most reliable procedure for detecting lymph node metastases [9]. Consequently, avoiding lymphadenectomy in high-risk groups rarely happens, leading to a range of expected side effects.

Attempts to improve the specificity of emerging diagnostic imaging tools have been made and could be incorporated into the nomograms. The mpMRI has the capacity to rank extracapsular extension (ECE) as a score, helping to decide the biopsy method—either transperineal systematic randomized biopsy (PI-RADS <2) or targeted biopsies (PI-RADS >3)—thereby improving diagnostic performance. Moreover, the mpMRI helped to increase the AUC for the Briganti-validated nomogram. Including ECE in the validated nomogram increased the AUC to 81%, which is consistent with findings from other researchers [10]. As a result, ECE should currently be considered the most important predictor of LNI at final pathology. These developments seem promising, and efforts to achieve prospective validation are needed to guide clinical practice.

To make decisions on upfront surgical treatment, one needs to consider a curative procedure and the minimal risk of microscopic lymph node involvement, aiming for definitive improvement in overall and cancer-specific survival. It is crucial to identify the best candidates for this procedure while considering the already described risk of complications it brings.

The PIVOT trial compared the beneficial effect of the prostatectomy procedure versus observation for different risk groups of patients with prostate cancer. With a median follow-up of 12.7 years, this trial showed an absolute difference in risk for death attributed to prostate cancer, favoring the surgical procedure by 4.0 percentage points (95% CI, −0.2 to 8.3; hazard ratio, 0.63; 95% CI, 0.39–1.02; P = 0.06). The median survival was 13.0 years with surgery and 12.4 years with observation. However, for overall survival, both low-risk and high-risk diseases showed only minimal absolute beneficial effects on survival, with 0.7 and 2.3%, respectively. In contrast, the intermediate-risk group had an absolute difference of 14.5% (95% CI, 2.8–25.6) [11].

These results should be interpreted with caution. The intermediate-risk group will likely have better overall survival outcomes with this approach, while observation remains a well-validated therapeutic option for the low-risk group (including non-clinically significant disease) [12]. However, observation should not be considered a therapeutic option for the high-risk group, even though the PIVOT trial did not identify a statistically significant beneficial effect on survival for the surgical arm over the observation arm for this group of patients. Instead, it should be interpreted that a surgical procedure for high-risk patients is not a suitable option and is as ineffective as merely monitoring the progression in these patients. These premises are supported by subsequent studies designed to evaluate the concurrent management of radiotherapy with and without hormonal therapy.

4. Risk groups for prostate cancer and definitive managements in localized disease

The NCCN guidelines define and classify five risk groups for prostate cancer [13]:

1. *Very low risk*: the patient has all of the following: cT1c, Grade Group 1, PSA < 10 ng/dL, fewer than 3 prostate biopsy fragments/cores positive, ≤50% cancer in each fragment/core, and PSA density < 0.15 ng/mL/g.

2. *Low risk*: the patient has cT1–cT2a, Grade Group 1, and PSA <10 ng/mL, with at least one variable from the very low-risk category missing.

3. *Intermediate risk*: the patient has cT2b–cT2c, Grade Group 2 or 3, and PSA 10–20 ng/mL. Additionally, this group may be separated into favorable and unfavorable subgroups according to whether ≥50% of biopsy cores are positive (e.g., ≥6 of 12 cores), having 2 of 3 variables, or having Grade Group 3.

4. *High risk*: the patient has cT3a, Grade Group 4 or Grade Group 5, and PSA >20 ng/mL, with only one of these criteria needing to be present.

5. *Very high risk*: these patients fall into the high-risk category but have at least one of the following: cT3b–cT4, Primary Gleason pattern 5, 2, or 3 high-risk features, or more than 4 cores with Grade Group 4 or 5.

Recommendations for non-surgical definitive treatments may be offered based on clinical trial data and valid sources according to the definitions used at the time the studies were designed. Therefore, referrals to intermediate-risk groups involve both favorable and unfavorable risk subgroups. Similarly, the high-risk prostate cancer group includes patients with very high-risk variables.

4.1 Intermediate-risk group

The definitive management of intermediate-risk prostate cancer can include a curative intention through prostatectomy. However, not all patients are good candidates for surgical procedures. Some may not accept the adverse effects profile, and others may have a low life expectancy. Therefore, definitive management through radiation could be an option.

The RTOG 9408 trial compared definitive radiotherapy (RT) with and without hormone treatment for T1b, T1c, T2a, or T2b prostate adenocarcinoma and a PSA level of 20 ng/mL or less. With a follow-up of 9.1 years, the use of short-term ADT (androgen deprivation therapy) before and during radiotherapy was associated with significantly decreased disease-specific mortality and increased overall survival [14]. However, these results have been inconsistent across prospective studies, particularly regarding overall survival [15]. A detrimental effect was reported in a meta-analysis that included retrospective studies, showing an increased risk of all-cause mortality by 12% (HR 1.12, 95% CI 1.01–1.12, $p = 0.04$) when ADT was added to radiotherapy [16]. Therefore, while radiotherapy is suggested to be effective, whether to add a short course of hormonotherapy remains an unresolved question.

4.2 High-risk group

The role of androgen deprivation therapy (ADT) for the high-risk population has been consistently shown to have a beneficial effect on survival. Studies such as RTOG 9202, 8531, and EORTC 22893 demonstrated improved overall survival, particularly in patients with a Gleason score of 7–10, with a cardiovascular safety profile and a longest median follow-up of 9.1 years. These studies, however, are heterogeneous in their definition of high risk and the duration of ADT (24–36 months) [17–19].

The NCCN guidelines currently propose the most precise definition for high risk, grouping both high-risk and very high-risk patients under the same therapeutic intention. While guidelines from the American Urological Association (AUA), European Association of Urology (EAU), American Society for Radiation Oncology (ASTRO), and National Comprehensive Cancer Network (NCCN) each have their definitions for "high-risk disease," it is essential to select those that consider cancer-specific and global mortality. The most appropriate guidelines incorporate all available variables to complete the risk classification for each center [20].

Currently, there is limited evidence supporting ADT combined with radiotherapy for less than 24 months. A study comparing 36 months versus 18 months of ADT combined with radiotherapy aimed to evaluate overall survival (OS) and quality of life (QoL) at 5 years. The 5-year OS rates were 91% (95% CI, 88–95%) for the 36-month group and 86% for the 18-month group (95% CI, 83–90%), with a p-value of 0.07. The research group concluded that 36 months of ADT is not superior to 18 months [21]. However, only about 25% of the cohort could be classified as a high-risk prostate cancer population.

The efficacy of adding abiraterone and prednisolone to androgen deprivation therapy (ADT) in high-risk localized prostate cancer was recently published. Patients with nodal involvement, or without node involvement but with stage T3 or T4 disease, Gleason score of 8–10, and prostate-specific antigen (PSA) concentration ≥40 ng/mL should receive abiraterone plus prednisone in addition to standard ADT and radiotherapy. This recommendation also applies to high-risk patients who relapse within ≤12 months of total ADT, have an interval of ≥12 months without treatment, and have a PSA concentration ≥4 ng/mL with a doubling time of <6 months, or a PSA concentration ≥20 ng/mL without evidence of metastatic disease.

Although median overall survival was not reached in both arms of the study, there was a reduction in the probability of death from all causes (HR 0.60, 95% CI 0.48–0.73, $p < 0.0001$), leading to approval for this treatment regimen in this setting [22].

For other outcomes, the incorporation of a brachytherapy (BT) boost to external beam radiotherapy (EBRT) showed superior 9-year biochemical failure-free survival (BFFS) rates and better local tumor control compared to EBRT alone. However, a general increase in late genitourinary (GU) toxicity was reported as a consequence [23]. This approach should be considered where available, with discussions with patients about the extended profile of potential side effects.

5. Emerging options in treatment and classification

Although the risk of biochemical failure and PSA persistence is higher after radical prostatectomy compared to other risk groups, some patients with a life expectancy of 10 years or higher are considered good candidates for surgical curative procedures. This therapeutic approach is primarily recommended in areas with limited resources [20], and the side effects profile should be clearly communicated to the patient. Perhaps, minimally invasive procedures could replace surgery in the future.

MRI-guided transurethral ultrasound ablation (TULSA) is an emerging image-guided therapy that maximizes the ability to treat localized prostate cancer while minimizing damage to the prostate. The ongoing CAPTAIN trial (NCT05027477) aims to define the role of this procedure compared to standard prostatectomy, with an estimated completion date in December 2034.

There are new commercially available protein-based biomarkers and biopsy-based multigene expression classifiers. However, none of these have undergone prospective validation, and no clinical decisions can currently be made based on these results [24]. Emerging data focuses on mutations associated with the androgen receptor (AR) pathway and sensitivity to androgenic suppressive therapy. SPOP mutations are most frequent in localized and metastatic prostate cancer, with ongoing studies assessing their predictive and prognostic value [25].

Recently, circulating DNA has gained traction in solid neoplasms, aiding in identifying targeted therapies and serving as a predictive and prognostic biomarker, particularly in lung and gynecological malignancies rather than prostate cancer. While liquid biopsies have been considered for metastatic or advanced disease, their role in localized prostate cancer remains unclear. In a prospective cohort where 28% had ISUP grade 3 and 57.1% had ISUP grade 4 or 5 localized prostate cancer, ctDNA from tumor cells *via* next-generation sequencing was not detected prior to surgery or at recurrence. The assay showed a sensitivity of 93% and specificity of 100% for detecting mutant cfDNA alleles. The authors concluded that this assay is less sensitive than PSA testing for measuring disease burden in localized prostate cancer [26].

Another research group conducted whole-genome sequencing of tumor-normal pairs in eight patients, where two patients had persistent ctDNA after prostatectomy, both of whom experienced early recurrence compared to those who did not [27].

6. Conclusions

Despite numerous attempts to incorporate liquid biopsies into the diagnosis and management of prostate cancer, they are not approved for this purpose. Currently, there is a lack of evidence to recommend their use in localized prostate neoplasms. Instead, significant advancements in diagnosis have been achieved by integrating validated diagnostic methods such as mpMRI and PET/CT imaging, which are crucial for accurate staging and guiding effective therapeutic strategies.

With the recent introduction of second-generation antiandrogens like Abiraterone for localized prostate cancer, circulating tumor DNA (ctDNA) could potentially be redirected to identify a subgroup of high-risk patients who would benefit from this therapy, similar to those in approved subgroups.

The oncological effectiveness of minimally invasive treatments compared to standard care is still being investigated. Current evidence supports radiotherapy, often combined with hormonal deprivation therapy, as the cornerstone of definitive treatment. Side effects profiles should be discussed synchronously during treatment, and the potential benefits of hormonal therapy beyond 24 months remain uncertain, as no prospective studies have directly compared 24 vs. 36 months of treatment. Shared decision-making with patients is crucial in such cases.

Ultimately, the appropriate staging and classification of early or localized prostate cancer should guide treatment decisions. Each risk group requires careful consideration of multiple variables before initiating definitive management, and decisions should ideally be made through multidisciplinary team discussions.

Conflict of interest

The authors declare no conflict of interest.

Appendices and nomenclature

NCI/SEER	National Cancer Institute/Surveillance, Epidemiology, and End Results
mpMRI	multiparametric magnetic resonance image
SCD	specific cancer death
ADT	androgen deprivation therapy
TULSA	MRI-guided transurethral ultrasound ablation
ctDNA	circulating tumor DNA
PET-CT	positron emission tomography-computed tomography scan
PSMA	prostatic specific membrane antigen
18F-DCFPyL	2-(3-{1-carboxy-5-[(6-[18F]fluoro-pyridine-3-carbonyl)-amino]-pentyl}-ureido)-pentanedioic acid

Author details

Sergio Contreras
Instituto Nacional de Ciencias Médicas y Nutrición "Salvador Zubirán" Tlalpan, Ciudad de México, Mexico

*Address all correspondence to: sergio.contrerasg@incmnsz.mx; sergiocongares@gmail.com

IntechOpen

© 2024 The Author(s). Licensee IntechOpen. This chapter is distributed under the terms of the Creative Commons Attribution License (http://creativecommons.org/licenses/by/4.0), which permits unrestricted use, distribution, and reproduction in any medium, provided the original work is properly cited.

References

[1] Wang L, Lu B, He M, Wang Y, Wang Z, Du L. Prostate cancer incidence and mortality: Global status and temporal trends in 89 countries from 2000 to 2019. Frontiers in Public Health. 2022;**10**:811044

[2] Shore ND. Current and future management of locally advanced and metastatic prostate cancer. Revista de Urología. 2020;**22**(3):110-123

[3] Rider JR, Sandin F, Andrén O, Wiklund P, Hugosson J, Stattin P. Long-term outcomes among noncuratively treated men according to prostate cancer risk category in a nationwide, population-based study. European Urology. 2013;**63**(1):88-96

[4] Szabo Z, Mena E, Rowe SP, et al. Initial evaluation of [(18)F]DCFPyL for prostate-specific membrane antigen (PSMA)-targeted PET imaging of prostate cancer. Molecular Imaging and Biology. 2015;**17**:565-574

[5] Madan RA, Mena E, Lindenberg L, Choyke PL. With new technology comes great responsibility: Prostate-specific membrane antigen imaging in recurrent prostate cancer. Journal of Clinical Oncology. 2022;**40**(26):3015-3019. DOI: 10.1200/JCO.22.00493

[6] Anttinen M, Ettala O, Malaspina S, Jambor I, Sandell M, Kajander S, et al. A prospective comparison of 18F-prostate-specific membrane antigen-1007 positron emission tomography computed tomography, whole-body 1.5 T magnetic resonance imaging with diffusion-weighted imaging, and single-photon emission computed tomography/computed tomography with traditional imaging in primary distant metastasis staging of prostate cancer (PROSTAGE). European Urology Oncology. 2021;**4**(4):635-644

[7] Hagens MJ, Luining WI, Jager A, Donswijk ML, Cheung Z, Wondergem M, et al. The diagnostic value of PSMA PET/CT in men with newly diagnosed unfavorable intermediate-risk prostate cancer. Journal of Nuclear Medicine. 2023;**64**(8):1238-1243

[8] Huang MM, Su ZT, Becker REN, Pavlovich CP, Partin AW, Allaf ME, et al. Complications after open and robot-assisted radical prostatectomy and association with postoperative opioid use: An analysis of data from the PREVENTER trial. BJU International. 2021;**127**(2):190-197

[9] Di Pierro GB, Salciccia S, Frisenda M, Tufano A, Sciarra A, Scarrone E, et al. Comparison of four validated nomograms (Memorial Sloan Kettering Cancer Center, Briganti 2012, 2017, and 2019) predicting lymph node invasion in patients with high-risk prostate cancer candidates for radical prostatectomy and extended pelvic lymph node dissection: Clinical experience and review of the literature. Cancers (Basel). 2023;**15**(6):1683

[10] Gandaglia G, Fossati N, Zaffuto E, Bandini M, Dell'Oglio P, Bravi CA, et al. Development and internal validation of a novel model to identify the candidates for extended pelvic lymph node dissection in prostate cancer. European Urology. 2017;**72**(4):632-640. DOI: 10.1016/j.eururo.2017.03.049

[11] Wilt TJ, Jones KM, Barry MJ, Andriole GL, Culkin D, Wheeler T, et al. Follow-up of prostatectomy versus observation for early prostate cancer. The New England Journal of Medicine. 2017;**377**(2):132-142

[12] Hamdy FC, Donovan JL, Lane JA, Metcalfe C, Davis M, Turner EL, et al. Fifteen-year outcomes after monitoring, surgery, or radiotherapy for prostate cancer. The New England Journal of Medicine. 2023;**388**(17):1547-1558

[13] Schaeffer EM, Srinivas S, Adra N, An Y, Barocas D, Bitting R, et al. Prostate cancer, version 4.2023, NCCN clinical practice guidelines in oncology. Journal of the National Comprehensive Cancer Network. 2023;**21**(10):1067-1096

[14] Jones CU, Hunt D, McGowan DG, Amin MB, Chetner MP, Bruner DW, et al. Radiotherapy and short-term androgen deprivation for localized prostate cancer. The New England Journal of Medicine. 2011;**365**(2):107-118

[15] Nabid A, Carrier N, Vigneault E, Van Nguyen T, Vavassis P, Brassard MA, et al. Androgen deprivation therapy and radiotherapy in intermediate-risk prostate cancer: A randomised phase III trial. European Journal of Cancer. 2021;**143**:64-74

[16] Chen J, Yuan Y, Fang M, Zhu Y, Sun X, Lou Y, et al. Androgen deprivation therapy and radiotherapy in intermediate-risk prostate cancer: A systematic review and meta-analysis. Frontiers in Endocrinology (Lausanne). 2023;**13**:1074540

[17] Pilepich MV, Winter K, Lawton CA, Krisch RE, Wolkov HB, Movsas B, et al. Androgen suppression adjuvant to definitive radiotherapy in prostate carcinoma--long-term results of phase III RTOG 85-31. International Journal of Radiation Oncology, Biology, Physics. 2005;**61**(5):1285-1290

[18] Bolla M, Van Tienhoven G, Warde P, Dubois JB, Mirimanoff RO, Storme G, et al. External irradiation with or without long-term androgen suppression for prostate cancer with high metastatic risk: 10-year results of an EORTC randomised study. The Lancet Oncology. 2010;**11**(11):1066-1073

[19] Bolla M, de Reijke TM, Van Tienhoven G, Van den Bergh AC, Oddens J, Poortmans PM, et al. Duration of androgen suppression in the treatment of prostate cancer. The New England Journal of Medicine. 2009;**360**(24):2516-2527

[20] Khauli R, Ferrigno R, Guimarães G, Bulbulan M, Uson Junior PLS, Salvajoli B, et al. Treatment of localized and locally advanced, high-risk prostate cancer: A report from the first prostate cancer consensus conference for developing countries. JCO Global Oncology. 2021;**7**:530-537

[21] Nabid A, Carrier N, Martin AG, Bahary JP, Lemaire C, Vass S, et al. Duration of androgen deprivation therapy in high-risk prostate cancer: A randomized phase III trial. European Urology. 2018;**74**(4):432-441

[22] Attard G, Murphy L, Clarke NW, Sachdeva A, Jones C, Hoyle A, et al. Abiraterone acetate plus prednisolone with or without enzalutamide for patients with metastatic prostate cancer starting androgen deprivation therapy: Final results from two randomised phase 3 trials of the STAMPEDE platform protocol. The Lancet Oncology. 2023;**24**(5):443-456

[23] Rodda S, Tyldesley S, Morris WJ, et al. ASCENDE-RT: An analysis of treatment-related morbidity for a randomized trial comparing a low-dose-rate brachytherapy boost with a dose-escalated external beam boost for high- and inter- mediate-risk prostate cancer. International Journal of Radiation Oncology, Biology, Physics. 2017;**98**:286-295

[24] Eggener SE, Rumble RB, Armstrong AJ, Morgan TM, Crispino T, Cornford P, et al. Molecular biomarkers in localized prostate cancer: ASCO guideline. Journal of Clinical Oncology. 2020;**38**(13):1474-1494

[25] Nakazawa M, Fang M, Marshall HC, Lotan TL, Isaacsson Velho P, Antonarakis ES. Clinical and genomic features of SPOP-mutant prostate cancer. The Prostate. 2022;**82**(2):260-268

[26] Hennigan ST, Trostel SY, Terrigino NT, Voznesensky OS, Schaefer RJ, Whitlock NC, et al. Low abundance of circulating tumor DNA in localized prostate cancer. JCO Global Oncology. 2019;**3**:PO.19.00176

[27] Lau E, McCoy P, Reeves F, Chow K, Clarkson M, Kwan EM, et al. Detection of ctDNA in plasma of patients with clinically localised prostate cancer is associated with rapid disease progression. Genome Medicine. 2020;**12**(1):72

Chapter 8

Surgical Methods to Improve Urinary Continence after Radical Robot-Assisted Prostatectomy: An Analysis of the Evidence Base of Meta-Analyses

Anushavan Papoyan, Marat Urmantsev, Peter Mironov and Ildar Lutfarakhmanov

Abstract

Currently, robot-assisted radical prostatectomy (PARP) allows for achieving excellent oncological results with a low complication rate and is the "gold standard" for extirpative treatment of prostate cancer. Post-prostatectomy incontinence is the most devastating complication, significantly affecting the physical activity, and social and psychological well-being of men, and therefore has a significant impact on quality of life regardless of cancer outcomes and sexual function, which may have a potential impact on the choice of PARP as a treatment option. In a number of randomized and non-randomized clinical trials, the new techniques were compared with standard PARP, and their results were summarized in systematic reviews and meta-analyses. The aim of this overview was to compare the functional outcomes of various modifications of RARP in order to obtain reliable results and create a basis for clinical guidelines. Systematic reviews and meta-analyses were searched using the PubMed system in the electronic databases Medline, Embase, Cochrane Library, Web of Science, and Google Scholar until January 2024. Thus, this overview of meta-analyses fills an important gap in knowledge about the efficacy of new PARP techniques to guide clinical practice and future research and provide a basis for clinical guidelines.

Keywords: prostate cancer, robot-assisted radical prostatectomy, urinary incontinence, systematic review, meta-analysis

1. Introduction

With the growing aging of the population and the popularization of early screening, the proportion of patients with localized prostate cancer has increased [1]. Today, this cancer is the second most common neoplasm in men, and one of the most frequently diagnosed in the world. In 2020, 1,414,259 new cases and 375,304 deaths were registered; over the two decades, a dramatic increase in morbidity and mortality is predicted to almost double [2].

In the early 2000s, Claude Abbou and Jochen Binder introduced robot-assisted radical prostatectomy (RARP) as a minimally invasive procedure [3, 4]. Currently, RARP can achieve excellent oncological results with a low complication rate and is the "gold standard" for extirpative treatment of prostate cancer.

Post-prostatectomy urinary incontinence is the most devastating complication, significantly affecting men's physical activity and social and psychological well-being, and therefore has a significant impact on quality of life regardless of cancer outcomes and sexual function, which may have a potential impact on the choice of RAPP as a treatment option. Urinary continence is a multifactorial process that encompasses demographic characteristics, anatomical and surgical aspects, surgeon's experience, and postoperative factors. Surgical technique is the only modifiable factor among them, and therefore the identification and development of the optimal operative technique probably affects the functional outcomes of RARP.

Because of the different surgical approaches, the aim of this overview was to compare the functional outcomes of various modifications of RARP in order to obtain reliable results and create a basis for clinical guidelines.

2. Methods

Systematic reviews and meta-analyses were searched using the PubMed system in the electronic databases Medline, Embase, Cochrane Library, Web of Science, and Google Scholar until January 2024. The search strategy included all possible combinations of the medical subject headings (MeSH) terms: prostate cancer/tumor/neoplasm; radical prostatectomy; postoperative complications; urinary continence/incontinence.

Systematic reviews were refined through a filtering process using the following criteria: (1) Participants were defined as adult men with prostate cancer who underwent RARP. (2) Interventions: bladder neck preservation; nerve-sparing; posterior reconstruction; Retzius-sparing; total reconstruction (3) Controls: conventional RARP. (4) Outcomes: The primary outcome was urinary continence/incontinence; the secondary outcome was the positive surgical margins (PSMs) status. Systematic reviews were excluded if: (1) The inclusion criteria were not met. (2) No outcomes of interest were reported. (4) Not written in English. Systematic reviews that met the exclusion criteria were excluded, even if they otherwise met the inclusion criteria.

Two reviewers (Anushavan Papoyan and Marat Urmantsev) independently screened the title, abstract, and keywords. The full text of any potentially relevant publication was retrieved for review, and systematic reviews were selected based on the criteria previously outlined. Any disagreements were resolved through open discussion and consultation with a third reviewer (Peter Mironov and Ildar Lutfarakhmanov). In all cases of missing or incomplete data, the corresponding authors were contacted, but no additional information was provided. The following data were extracted including: first author, database(s) used and search deadline, surgical approach, technique proposed, baseline characteristics of the trials, the overall number of patients who underwent the proposed technique or control, outcomes of interest, and evidence gaps.

Using the electronic search strategy, a total of 24 systematic reviews were considered suitable for the current overview, of which 21 meta-analyses were finally included. This overview included 12 full-text report meta-analyses [5–16] and nine meta-analyses [17–25] available as abstracts only, so we recognize the importance of selective reporting bias. We did not include the results of two systematic reviews [26, 27] because the authors did not conduct a meta-analysis of the data. Also, we did not include the results of one meta-analysis [28] because the authors have demonstrated an association between NS and continence during non-RARP surgery.

3. Analysis of the evidence base for modifications of surgical techniques

Table 1 provides an overview of meta-analyses of the effects of different surgical techniques in optimizing the recovery of urinary continence after PARP.

3.1 Bladder neck preservation (BNP)

The technique of BNP has evolved from a better knowledge of the anatomy and physiology of the mechanisms involved in urinary continence. First introduced in 1992, BNP has been proposed as a method to accelerate continence recovery after radical prostatectomy.

The first meta-analysis [5] comparing BNP and non-BNP approaches demonstrated that BNP surgery improved early recovery and overall long-term urinary continence outcomes and was effective in eradicating prostate cancer without increasing the recurrence rate.

Meta-analysis [6] demonstrated that the BNP technique during RARP improved both short-term and long-term urinary continence recovery without compromising the oncologic outcomes. The odds ratio (OR) for continence rate at 12 months was 2.03 (95% confidence interval [CI] 1.10–3.74), which seemed to be higher than that reported previously [5]. These observations suggested that the favorable effect of the BNP technique might be more effective when it is performed as a part of RARP.

3.2 Nerve-sparing (NS)

Recent anatomical findings have led to the idea that the NS technique leads to earlier urinary continence recovery after radical prostatectomy.

Meta-analysis [7] showed that the technique of intrafascial NS-RARP was associated with an earlier recovery of urinary continence, with statistically significant differences at 1, 3, and 6 months. This advantage, however, was not present at 12 months. Authors only detected that the retropubic approach was associated with a lower continence rate as compared with laparoscopic and robot-assisted radical prostatectomy; however, since only one study was included in this analysis, this result may be biased.

Meta-analysis [8] indicated that NS-RARP was feasible during surgeries and was beneficial for the long-term (12 months after surgeries) urination continence recovery of high-risk patients, and was associated with better oncological outcomes. However, due to interference factors, it is not clear whether this advantage is caused by NS itself.

3.3 Posterior reconstruction

The posterior reconstruction technique was originally proposed to improve the urinary continence recovery after retropubic radical prostatectomy.

Meta-analysis [17] showed that restoration of the posterior aspect of the rhabdosphincter improved continence recovery up to 90 days after surgery, while the

Technique proposed	First author	Database(s)/Deadline	Surgical approach	Trials selected; patients: cases/ controls	Urination status	Evidence gaps
Bladder neck preservation	Ma X [5]	PubMed, Ovid Medline, Embase, CBM, Cochrane Library/February 2016	Open/ Lap/ RARP	• 13 studies: 2 RCTs, 6 prospective, 5 retrospective • 2284 patients: 1130/ 1154	Continence (OR): • > 12 mo: 3.99; 1.94–8.21; < 0.001	• Lack of prospective studies • Small sample sizes • Language restrictions • Short follow-up time
	Kim JW [6]	PubMed, Medline, Embase, Cochrane Library/ May 2019	RARP	• 4 studies: 2 prospective, 2 retrospective • 2607 patients: 1880/727	Continence (OR): • 3–4 mo: 2.88; 1.52–5.48; 0,001 • 12 mo: 2.03; 1.10–3.74; 0.020 • 24 mo: 3.23; 1.13–9.20; 0.030	• Non-RCT observational studies • Continence recovery evaluation • Individual surgeon factors • Language restrictions
Nerve-sparing	Wang X [7]	PubMed/October 2017	Open/ Lap/ RARP	• 6 studies, 1 RARP: 1 RCT, 5 observational • 1558 patients: 747/ 841	Continence (OR): • 4 wk.: 3.26; 1.00–10.64; 0.050 • 12 wk.: 1.82; 1.18–2.82; 0.007 • 24 wk.: 2.19; 1.43–3.34; < 0.001 • 48 wk.: 1.33; 0.83–2.13; 0.230	• Lack of RCTs
	Liu Y [8]	Pubmed, Cochrane Library, Web of Science, Embase/December 2022	RARP	• 3 studies: 1 prospective, 2 retrospective • 1370 patients: 150/ 1220	Continence, Non-NS vs. NS (RR): • 48 wk.: 0.46; 0.22–0.96; 0.045	• Only cohort studies • Loss of follow-up • Heterogeneity in the techniques and postoperative rehabilitation protocols
Posterior reconstruction	Grasso AA [17]	Medline, Embase, Scopus, Web of Science/June 2015	Open/ Lap/ RARP	• 21 studies: 3 RCTs, 5 prospective, 13 retrospective • 3600 patients: 2080/1520	Continence (RR): • 3–7 d: 1.07; 0.75–1.51 • 30 d: 1.69; 0.46–6.27 • 90 d: 1.48; 0.41–5.32 • 180 d: 1.13; 0.70–1.82	• Language restrictions

Technique proposed	First author	Database(s)/Deadline	Surgical approach	Trials selected; patients: cases/controls	Urination status	Evidence gaps
	Cui J [9]	PubMed, Embase, Cochrane Library, Ovid, Web of Science/June 2016	Open/Lap/RARP	• 19 studies: 2 RCTs, 17 cohort • 2855 patients: 1684/1171	Continence (RR): • 1–4 d: 3.70; 2.34–5.84; < 0.001 • 7–14 d: 1.28; 0.98–1.67; 0.073 • 28–42 d: 1.63; 1.26–2.10; < 0.001 • 90 d: 1.28; 1.06–1.55; 0.009 • 180 d: 1.14; 1.00–1.30; 0.044 • 360 d: 1.23; 1.03–1.48; 0.021	Different: • Study designs • Surgical technics • Continence evaluation • Number of patients treated Language restrictions
	Rosenberg JE [10]	Cochrane Library, Medline, Embase, Web of Science, Scopus, Global Index Medicus, ClinicalTrials, WHO ICTRP/March 2021	RARP	• 6 RCTs • 842 patients: 437/405	Continence (RR): • 1 wk.: 1.25; 0.90–1.73 • 12 wk.: 0.98; 0.84–1.14 • 24 wk.: 1.01; 0.97–1.05 • 48 wk.: 1.02; 0.98–1.07	Different: • Continence evaluation • Surgical methods • Surgeon experience
Retzius-sparing	Dirie NI [11]	Web of Science, PubMed, EMBase, Cochrane Library, Google Scholar/September 2017	RARP	• 4 studies: 1 RCT, 1 prospective, 2 retrospective • 500 patients: 250/250	Continence (OR), 1 mo: • Total: 3.53; 1.48–8.40; 0.004 • 0 pads: 4.07; 2.03–8.14; < 0.001	• Limitations of observational studies • Short follow-up time • Smaller data
	Checcucci E [18]	Medline, Embase, Cochrane Library/2020	RARP	• 7 studies: 2 RCTs, 2 prospective, 3 retrospective • 451 patients: 220/231	Continence (OR): • 4 wk.: 2.54; 1.16–5.53; 0.020 • 12 wk.: 3.86; 2.23–6.68; < 0.001 • 24 wk.: 3.61; 1.88–6.91; 0.001 • 48 wk.: 7.29; 1.89–28.13; 0.004	Not available

Technique proposed	First author	Database(s)/Deadline	Surgical approach	Trials selected; patients: cases/controls	Urination status	Evidence gaps
	Jiang YL [12]	PubMed, Embase, Cochrane Library/2019	RARP	• 7 studies: 2 RCTs, 3 prospective, 2 retrospective • 803 patients: 395/408	Continence (OR): • 2.86; 1.94–4.20; < 0.001	• Lack of RCTs • Surgeon experience representative • Not adequate follow-up time • Patients heterogeneity
	Phukan C [19]	PubMed/Medline, Cochrane Library/January 2018	RARP	• 6 studies: 2 RCTs, 4 observational	Continence (RR): • 4 wk.: 1.72; 1.27–2.32; < 0.001 • 12 wk.: 1.39; 1.03–1.88; 0.030	Not available
	Rosenberg JE [13]	Cochrane Library, Medline, Embase, Web of Science, Scopus, Global Index Medicus, ClinicalTrials, WHO ICTRP/June 2020	RARP	• 5 RCTs • 571 patients	Continence (RR): • 1 wk.: 1.74; 1.41–2.14 • 12 wk.: 1.33; 1.06–1.62 • 24 wk.: 1.09; 0.99–1.20 • 48 wk.: 1.01; 0.97–1.04	• Lack of clinical and methodologic details • Surgeon experience and learning curve • Performance bias
	Tai TE [20]	March 2019	RARP	• 2 RCTs, 4 observational	Incontinence (OR): • 4 wk.: 0.30; < 0.001 • 48 wk.: 0.25; < 0.001	Not available
	Xu JN [14]	Medline/PubMed, Cochrane Library, EMBASE, Web of Science/January 2021	RARP	• 12 studies: 4 RCTs, 6 prospective, 2 retrospective • 2379 patients: 1148/1231	Continence (OR): • ≤ 1 mo: 5.72; 3.56–9.19; < 0,001 • 3 mo: 6.44; 4.50–9.22; < 0.001 • 6 mo: 8.68; 4.01–18.82; < 0.001 • 12 mo: 2.37; 1.20–4.07; 0.010	• Heterogeneity of urine control outcome • Lack of long-term survival data

Technique proposed	First author	Database(s)/Deadline	Surgical approach	Trials selected; patients: cases/controls	Urination status	Evidence gaps
	Barakat B [21]	PubMed, Medline, EMBASE, Cochrane Library/March 2021	RARP	• 10 studies: 4 RCTs, 6 prospective • Not available	Continence (OR): • 1 wk.: 1.81; 1.26–2.60 • 12 wk.: 1.57; 0.69–3.58 • 24 wk.: 1.22; 0.89–1.66 • 48 wk.: 1.14; 0.98–1.32	Not available
	Chung DY [15]	PubMed, EMBASE, Cochrane Library/August 2021	RARP	• 5 studies: 3 RCTs, 2 retrospective • 573 patients: 280/293	Incontinence (OR): • 4 wk.: 0.28; 0.16–0.47; < 0.001 • 12 wk.: 0.31; 0.18–0.53; < 0.001 • 24 wk.: 0.29; 0.17–0.51; < 0.001 • 48 wk.: 0.64; 0.35–1.18; 0.150	• Lack of RCTs • Different surgeon experience and surgical techniques
	Liu J [22]	Not available	RARP	Not available	Incontinence (OR): • 1 wk.: 0.40; 0.20–0.77; < 0.001 • 4 wk.: 0.17; 0.10–0.29; < 0.001 • 12 wk.: 0.18; 0.09–0.36; < 0.001 • 24 wk.: 0.26; 0.15–0.46; < 0.001 • 48 wk.: 0.50; 0.28–0.89; 0.020	Not available
	Nunes-Silva I [23]	Medline/PubMed, Cochrane Library	RARP	• 4 retrospective studies • 87 patients	Continence (OR): • 4.36; 1.7–11.17	Limitations of cohort studies
	O'Connor-Cordova MA [24]	February 2023	RARP	• 17 studies • 2751 patients: 1221/1530	Continence (OR): • 1 mo: 4.57; 1.32–15.77 • 3 mo: 2.93; 1.57–5.46 • 12 mo: 4.37; 1.97–9.73	Not available

Technique proposed	First author	Database(s)/Deadline	Surgical approach	Trials selected; patients: cases/ controls	Urination status	Evidence gaps
Total reconstruction	Ficarra V [25]	Medline, Embase, Web of Science/August 2011	RARP	• 17 comparative studies, 17 clinical series >100 cases	Incontinence (OR): • 3 mo: 0.76; 0.040	Not available
	Wu YP [16]	PubMed, Embase, Web of Science/November 2017	RARP	• 10 studies: 5 RCTs, 2 prospective, 3 retrospective • 2922 patients: 2052/ 870	Continence (OR): • 1 wk.: 2.76; 1.58–4.84; < 0.001 • 2 wk.: 2.57; 1.74–3.80; < 0.001 • 4 wk.: 2.61; 1.56–4.38; < 0.001 • 12 wk.: 4.33; 2.01–9.33; < 0.001 • 24 wk.: 3.83; 1.54–9.55; 0.004 • 52 wk.: 4.10; 1.80–9.38; < 0.001	Different: • Study design • Surgical tec hnique • Urinary continence d definition

Data are presented (if available) as follows: odds ratio (OR) or risk ratio (RR); 95% confidence interval; p level.
Note. ICTRP, International Clinical Trials Registry Platform; Lap, laparoscopic radical prostatectomy; Open, retropubic radical prostatectomy; WHO, World Health Organization.

Table 1.
Review of the effect of surgical techniques on urinary continence after RARP.

continence rate at 180 days was not clinically affected. Statistically significantly lower anastomotic leakage rates were described after posterior reconstruction, and there were no differences in PSM rates.

Meta-analysis [9] included patients who underwent radical prostatectomy with posterior reconstruction, anterior reconstruction, anterior suspension, pelvic floor reconstruction, and total reconstruction modifications. Treatment of patients with posterior reconstruction improved the urinary continence rate at 0–4, 28–42, 90, 180, and 360 days after surgery.

Cochrane meta-analysis [10] found evidence that posterior reconstruction may result in improved continence 1 week after catheter removal but may result in little to no difference after 3 and 12 months after surgery (low-certainty evidence) and also probably does not 6 months after surgery (moderate-certainty evidence). Based on the available evidence, posterior reconstruction probably results in little to no difference in serious adverse events (moderate-certainty evidence). Posterior reconstruction may also result in little to no difference in PSMs and biochemical recurrence at 12 months after surgery compared to no posterior reconstruction (low-certainty evidence).

3.4 Retzius-sparing (RS)

The introduction of robotic surgery has contributed to the development of a new approach to radical prostatectomy, the so-called RS-RARP.

Meta-analysis [11] indicated that the RS technique, as opposed to the conventional anterior approach, was safe and feasible and was associated with an earlier recovery of urinary continence after the surgery, while PSM rates were similar in both groups.

Meta-analysis [18] summarized the current evidence on RS-RARP and compared its oncological, peri-operative, and functional outcomes with those of standard retropubic RARP. Analysis has confirmed that RS-RARP was associated with a faster recovery of continence. One caveat might be the higher rates of PSMs, probably related to an expected learning curve.

Meta-analysis [12] found that RS-RARP provided a better recovery of postoperative continence than non-RS-RARP. The perioperative outcomes (PSMs, complications, blood loss, and operative time) were comparable for the two groups.

Meta-analysis [19] of functional and oncological outcomes of RS-RARP and conventional RARP showed that RS-RARP was associated with better early continence rates ($\leq$ 1 month) (moderate quality evidence) and at 3 months (low-quality evidence). Based on very low-quality evidence, RS-RARP did not alter 6- and 12-month continence rates, as well as PSM rates.

Cochrane meta-analysis [13] represented the most rigorous and up-to-date systematic review on the question of RS-RARP. The quality of evidence, which ranged from moderate to very low. Indicated that RS-RARP resulted in better urinary continence recovery than conventional RARP up to 6 months after surgery. Downsides of RS-RARP were higher PSM rates.

Meta-analysis [20] revealed that RS-RARP had superior functional outcomes of urinary continence in the first month and 12th month and equivalent complication rates, but significantly higher PSM rates as compared with conventional RARP.

Meta-analysis [14] showed that the urinary continence recovery rates of the RS-RARP group were significantly higher than those of the conventional RARP group up to 12 months after surgery. In addition, the RS-RARP group had significantly higher PSM rates in the anterior site.

Meta-analysis [21] revealed that immediate continence recovery was higher and significantly advantageous for RS-RARP. Continence recovery also tended to be higher at 3 and 6 months. The urinary continence recovery at 12 months was similar in both groups. Meta-analysis showed PSM rates were statistically significantly higher following RS-RARP as compared with standard RARP, and there was no significant difference concerning the major complication rates.

Meta-analysis [15] showed that RS-RARP was superior to conventional RARP in early continence recovery, regardless of the postoperative period. However, there was no significant difference in the recovery of late continence after 12 months. Also, RS-RARP showed a relatively high PSM rate in locally advanced prostate cancer.

Meta-analysis [22] found that RS-RARP had better postoperative continence recovery than conventional RARP. There were also no significant differences in operation time, intraoperative blood loss, length of stay, PSMs, and complications.

Meta-analysis [23] showed that the RS-RARP approach had the potential to positively impact continence function in salvage surgery.

Meta-analysis [24] suggested that RS-RARP was safe and feasible. There were statistical differences in terms of continence recovery at 1 month, as well as at 3 months after RS-RARP as compared with conventional RARP. Meta-analysis revealed that overall PSM rates were not different following RS-RARP, as well as biochemical recurrence, estimated blood loss, length of stay, operation time, and complications.

3.5 Total reconstruction

The method of total reconstruction combines two important components: anterior and posterior reconstruction.

Meta-analysis [25] identified that posterior musculofascial reconstruction with or without anterior reconstruction was associated with a small advantage in urinary continence recovery 1 month after surgery. The only total reconstruction technique was associated with an advantage in urinary continence recovery 3 months after surgery.

Meta-analysis [16] demonstrated statistically significant differences in favor of the total reconstruction technique for urinary continence recovery. Total reconstruction was associated with an advantage for urinary continence recovery up to 52 weeks after surgery. No significant differences were observed for PSM rates.

4. Quality of evidence

There is an opinion that, in the experienced hands, most patients completely restore urinary continence after RARP without the need for special reconstructive techniques [29]. The two main surgical strategies are anatomical dissection of the bladder neck with a nerve-sparing attitude. However, some meta-analyses have suggested little difference in the return of continence when compared BNP with conventional RARP and the increased risk of PSMs. Nerve-sparing appears to be the most important aspect of RAPP, but this method may not be feasible for patients with locally advanced cancer. Although the results of meta-analyses have shown the benefits of RS-PARP in functional outcomes, this technique has limitations and cannot be used in all patients with cancer, including those with a large prostate volume. Since robotic platforms are not available in many urologic clinics, these modifications can

Surgical technique	Level of evidence
Bladder neck preservation	1a
Nerve-sparing	1b
Posterior reconstruction	1a
Retzius-sparing	1a
Total reconstruction	1b

Table 2.
Evidence base of surgical techniques to improve the urinary continence recovery after RARP.

possibly be adopted for use in retropubic or laparoscopic approaches. Results of meta-analysis demonstrated a significant advantage in favor of total reconstruction in terms of both short- and long-term urinary continence recoveries. However, methodological factors need to be taken into account when interpreting the cumulative results.

Table 2 summarizes the evidence for the effectiveness of various surgical techniques to optimize the continence recovery after RARP. There is a high level of evidence for the preservation of the sphincter mechanism and for the reconstruction of supporting structures.

5. Limitations

Although results from systematic reviews and meta-analyses present the best available evidence, some potential drawbacks should be mentioned. The first concern is related to the nature of non-randomized observational studies with inherent limitations such as selection bias. Second, continence recovery was not properly evaluated in all treated cases. Third, the impossibility of controlling for individual surgeon factors, such as surgical techniques and experience level. Fourth, short follow-up time and marked heterogeneity for several continuous variables have influenced the confidence of results to varying degrees. Fifth, the postoperative rehabilitation protocols for continence were absent, which could also be an issue when assessing postoperative results. Finally, only articles published in English were included, and individual data were not available for each meta-analysis.

6. Conclusions

To our knowledge, this is the only original overview of the available systematic reviews of reconstructive methods to improve urinary continence recovery with mixed results. Most meta-analyses showed a common result regarding the superiority of early recovery of urinary continence in modified techniques of RARP. However, compared with conventional RARP, late continence recovery and PSM rates are controversial. Our overview fills an important knowledge gap about the effectiveness of new RARP techniques to guide clinical practice and future research. The findings of this overview will contribute to the refinement and dissemination of the standardized approach to RARP and provide a basis for clinical guidelines.

Author details

Anushavan Papoyan[1†], Marat Urmantsev[1†], Peter Mironov[2†] and
Ildar Lutfarakhmanov[3*†]

1 Department of Urology and Oncology, Bashkir State Medical University, Russia

2 Bashkir State Medical University, Ufa, Republic of Bashkortostan, Russia

3 Department of Anesthesiology and Intensive Care, Bashkir State Medical University, Russia

*Address all correspondence to: an-rean@bashgmu.ru

† These authors contributed equally.

IntechOpen

© 2024 The Author(s). Licensee IntechOpen. This chapter is distributed under the terms of the Creative Commons Attribution License (http://creativecommons.org/licenses/by/4.0), which permits unrestricted use, distribution, and reproduction in any medium, provided the original work is properly cited.

References

[1] Siegel RL, Miller KD, Fuchs HE, Jemal A. Cancer statistics, 2022. CA: A Cancer Journal for Clinicians. 2022; **72**(1):7-33. DOI: 10.3322/caac.21708

[2] Sung H, Ferlay J, Siegel RL, Laversanne M, Soerjomataram I, Jemal A, et al. Global cancer statistics 2020: GLOBOCAN estimates of incidence and mortality worldwide for 36 cancers in 185 countries. CA: A Cancer Journal for Clinicians. 2021; **71**(3):209-249. DOI: 10.3322/caac.21660

[3] Abbou CC, Hoznek A, Salomon L, Olsson LE, Lobontiu A, Saint F, et al. Laparoscopic radical prostatectomy with a remote controlled robot. The Journal of Urology. 2001;**165**(6 Pt 1):1964-1966. DOI: 10.1097/00005392-200106000-00027

[4] Binder J, Jones J, Bentas W, Wolfram M, Bräutigam R, Probst M, et al. Roboterunterstützte Laparoskopie in der Urologie. Radikale Prostatektomie und rekonstruktive retroperitoneale Eingriffe [robot-assisted laparoscopy in urology. Radical prostatectomy and reconstructive retroperitoneal interventions]. Der Urologe: Ausg A. 2002;**41**(2):144-149. German. DOI: 10.1007/s00120-002-0178-2

[5] Ma X, Tang K, Yang C, Wu G, Xu N, Wang M, et al. Bladder neck preservation improves time to continence after radical prostatectomy: A systematic review and meta-analysis. Oncotarget. 2016;**7**(41):67463-67475. DOI: 10.18632/oncotarget.11997

[6] Kim JW, Kim DK, Ahn HK, Jung HD, Lee JY, Cho KS. Effect of bladder neck preservation on long-term urinary continence after robot-assisted laparoscopic prostatectomy: A systematic review and meta-analysis. Journal of Clinical Medicine. 2019;**8**(12): 2068. DOI: 10.3390/jcm8122068

[7] Wang X, Wu Y, Guo J, Chen H, Weng X, Liu X. Intrafascial nerve-sparing radical prostatectomy improves patients' postoperative continence recovery and erectile function: A pooled analysis based on available literatures. Medicine (Baltimore). 2018;**97**(29): e11297. DOI: 10.1097/MD.0000000000011297

[8] Liu Y, Deng XZ, Qin J, Wen Z, Jiang Y, Huang J, et al. Erectile function, urinary continence and oncologic outcomes of neurovascular bundle sparing robot-assisted radical prostatectomy for high-risk prostate cancer: A systematic review and meta-analysis. Frontiers in Oncology. 2023;**13**: 1161544. DOI: 10.3389/fonc.2023.1161544

[9] Cui J, Guo H, Li Y, Chen S, Zhu Y, Wang S, et al. Pelvic floor reconstruction after radical prostatectomy: A systematic review and meta-analysis of different surgical techniques. Scientific Reports. 2017;**7**(1):2737. DOI: 10.1038/s41598-017-02991-8

[10] Rosenberg JE, Jung JH, Lee H, Lee S, Bakker CJ, Dahm P. Posterior musculofascial reconstruction in robotic-assisted laparoscopic prostatectomy for the treatment of clinically localized prostate cancer. Cochrane Database of Systematic Reviews. 2021;**8**(8): CD013677. DOI: 10.1002/14651858.CD013677.pub2

[11] Dirie NI, Pokhrel G, Guan W, Mumin MA, Yang J, Masau JF, et al. Is Retzius-sparing robot-assisted radical prostatectomy associated with better functional and oncological outcomes? Literature review and meta-analysis.

Asian Journal of Urology. 2019;**6**(2): 174-182. DOI: 10.1016/j.ajur.2018.02.001

[12] Jiang YL, Zheng GF, Jiang ZP, Zhen-Li ZXL, Zhou J, Ye CH, et al. Comparison of Retzius-sparing robot-assisted laparoscopic radical prostatectomy vs standard robot-assisted radical prostatectomy: A meta-analysis. BMC Urology. 2020;**20**(1):114. DOI: 10.1186/s12894-020-00685-4

[13] Rosenberg JE, Jung JH, Edgerton Z, Lee H, Lee S, Bakker CJ, et al. Retzius-sparing versus standard robotic-assisted laparoscopic prostatectomy for the treatment of clinically localized prostate cancer. Cochrane Database of Systematic Reviews. 2020;**8**(8):CD013641. DOI: 10.1002/14651858.CD013641.pub2

[14] Xu JN, Xu ZY, Yin HM. Comparison of Retzius-sparing robot-assisted radical prostatectomy vs. conventional robot-assisted radical prostatectomy: An up-to-date meta-analysis. Frontiers in Surgery. 2021;**8**:738421. DOI: 10.3389/fsurg.2021.738421

[15] Chung DY, Jung HD, Kim DK, Lee MH, Lee SW, Paick S, et al. Outcomes of Retzius-sparing versus conventional robot-assisted radical prostatectomy: A KSER update series systematic review and meta-analysis. PLoS One. 2022;**17**(5):e0268182. DOI: 10.1371/journal.pone.0268182

[16] Wu YP, Xu N, Wang ST, Chen SH, Lin YZ, Li XD, et al. The efficacy and feasibility of total reconstruction versus nontotal reconstruction of the pelvic floor on short-term and long-term urinary continence rates after radical prostatectomy: A meta-analysis. World Journal of Surgical Oncology. 2017;**15**(1): 228. DOI: 10.1186/s12957-017-1296-z

[17] Grasso AA, Mistretta FA, Sandri M, Cozzi G, De Lorenzis E, Rosso M, et al. Posterior musculofascial reconstruction after radical prostatectomy: An updated systematic review and a meta-analysis. BJU International. 2016;**118**(1):20-34. DOI: 10.1111/bju.13480

[18] Checcucci E, Veccia A, Fiori C, Amparore D, Manfredi M, Di Dio M, et al. Retzius-sparing robot-assisted radical prostatectomy vs the standard approach: A systematic review and analysis of comparative outcomes. BJU International. 2020;**125**(1):8-16. DOI: 10.1111/bju.14887

[19] Phukan C, Mclean A, Nambiar A, Mukherjee A, Somani B, Krishnamoorthy R, et al. Retzius sparing robotic assisted radical prostatectomy vs. conventional robotic assisted radical prostatectomy: A systematic review and meta-analysis. World Journal of Urology. 2020;**38**(5):1123-1134. DOI: 10.1007/s00345-019-02798-4

[20] Tai TE, Wu CC, Kang YN, Wu JC. Effects of Retzius sparing on robot-assisted laparoscopic prostatectomy: A systematic review with meta-analysis. Surgical Endoscopy. 2020;**34**(9): 4020-4029. DOI: 10.1007/s00464-019-07190-2

[21] Barakat B, Othman H, Gauger U, Wolff I, Hadaschik B, Rehme C. Retzius sparing radical prostatectomy versus robot-assisted radical prostatectomy: Which technique is more beneficial for prostate cancer patients (MASTER study)? A systematic review and meta-analysis. European Urology Focus. 2022; **8**(4):1060-1071. DOI: 10.1016/j.euf.2021.08.003

[22] Liu J, Zhang J, Yang Z, Liu Q, Zhang W, Qing Z, et al. Comparison of Retzius-sparing and conventional robot-assisted laparoscopic radical prostatectomy regarding continence and sexual function: An updated

meta-analysis. Prostate Cancer and Prostatic Diseases. 2022;**25**(1):47-54. DOI: 10.1038/s41391-021-00459-5

[23] Nunes-Silva I, Hidaka AK, Glina FPA, Hayashi RM, Glina S. Can salvage Retzius-sparing robotic-assisted radical prostatectomy improve continence outcomes? A systematic review and meta-analysis study. World Journal of Urology. 2023;**41**(9): 2311-2317. DOI: 10.1007/s00345-023-04505-w

[24] O'Connor-Cordova MA, Macías AGO, Sancen-Herrera JP, Altamirano-Lamarque F, Vargas Del Toro A, Peddinani BK, et al. Surgical and functional outcomes of Retzius-sparing robotic-assisted radical prostatectomy versus conventional robotic-assisted radical prostatectomy in patients with biopsy-confirmed prostate cancer. Are outcomes worth it? Systematic review and meta-analysis. The Prostate. 2023; **83**(15):1395-1414. DOI: 10.1002/pros.24604

[25] Ficarra V, Novara G, Rosen RC, Artibani W, Carroll PR, Costello A, et al. Systematic review and meta-analysis of studies reporting urinary continence recovery after robot-assisted radical prostatectomy. European Urology. 2012; **62**(3):405-417. DOI: 10.1016/j.eururo.2012.05.045

[26] Mason JB, Hatch L, Dall C, Kowalczyk KJ. Salvage Retzius-sparing radical prostatectomy: A review of complications, functional outcomes, and oncologic outcomes. Current Oncology. 2022;**29**(12):9733-9743. DOI: 10.3390/curroncol29120764

[27] Smolski M, Esler RC, Turo R, Collins GN, Oakley N, Brough R. Bladder neck sparing in radical prostatectomy. Indian Journal of Urology. 2013;**29**(4): 338-344. DOI: 10.4103/0970-1591.120118

[28] Reeves F, Preece P, Kapoor J, Everaerts W, Murphy DG, Corcoran NM, et al. Preservation of the neurovascular bundles is associated with improved time to continence after radical prostatectomy but not long-term continence rates: Results of a systematic review and meta-analysis. European Urology. 2015;**68**(4):692-704. DOI: 10.1016/j.eururo.2014.10.020

[29] Sessa F, Nicoletti R, Pecoraro A, Polverino P, Rivetti A, Conte FL, et al. Urinary continence recovery after robotic radical prostatectomy without anterior or posterior reconstruction: Experience from a tertiary referral center. Journal of Clinical Medicine. 2023;**12**(4):1358. DOI: 10.3390/jcm12041358

Chapter 9

Prostate Cancer in the Sub-Saharan Region: Care, Management and Challenges for Upgrade

Ditsapelo M. McFarland and William M. Baratedi

Abstract

Prostate cancer (PCa) has been cited as the leading cancer in men in sub-Saharan Africa (SSA). Published data from a few registries in SSA suggest that the rates are still rising. Men In SSA are reported to be at higher risk of the disease, and are about twice as likely to die from prostate cancer than white men. Despite the achievement to reduce the incidence of PCa, globally, very little success has been reported in SSA. This study aimed to examine the status of PCa in SSA and describe its care, management and challenges. Data supporting this study were obtained through extensive internet search of articles, using specific search terns. The findings indicated that patients with PCa in SSA normally present for management at advanced stage of the disease. It is suggested that this could be due to lack of knowledge, insufficiently staffed facilities, perceptions by men toward PCa, and tests for the condition which are uncomfortable and do not conform to their culture. The search revealed challenges relating to health care system and socio-economic factors. There is a need to increase the knowledge on PCa among men in SSA, as well as for sufficient staffing and promotion of men-friendly services.

Keywords: prostate cancer, prostate care, prostate palliative, prostate perceptions, sub Saharan Africa

1. Introduction

Sub-Saharan Africa (SSA) is part of the African continent that lies south of the Sahara Desert excluding Sudan [1]. The region is one of the poorest in the world. It lags in development compared to the rest of the world despite much significant progress made in the past decades. Many populations in the region still experience high levels of poverty, food insecurity, poor infrastructural development with insufficient institutional capacity and environmental degradation [2]. Other challenges in the region are shortage of finance and exponential population growth [3]. Studies have noted that the world is expected to reach a population growth rate of 2.44% by 2050 and half of this will occur in Africa, accrediting it to having the fastest growing population [4]. Some countries are still grappling with high rates of communicable diseases like tuberculosis (TB) and the human immune-deficiency virus (HIV) and acquired immune deficiency syndrome (AIDS) which have reduced the life expectancy of their citizens [5]. SSA has for many decades been struggling with communicable diseases, but in recent years, a significant success has been realized, though the efforts on these are seemingly being reversed by the emergence of the non-communicable diseases which include cancers [6]. The authors' objective is to examine the current situation of prostate cancer (PCa) in sub-Saharan Africa and further describe how the region is managing the condition among the challenges that exist. Furthermore, recommendations will be proposed for governments to initiate in order to curb the increasing incidences of PCa. To achieve this, Data supporting this study were achieved through an extensive internet search of articles published not more than 12 years ago. These were from PubMed, EBSCOHOST, MedlinePlus, American Cancer Society (ACS), BioMedical Central (BMC), Google scholar, and National Comprehensive Cancer Network (NCCN).

2. State of prostate cancer in SSA

The SSA region is experiencing a rapid epidemiologic transition which is characterized by disease burden profiles shifting from the traditional communicable diseases like tuberculosis, malaria, AIDS, measles, and scabies, to the growing incidences and prevalences of non-communicable diseases (NCD) which include the cardiovascular conditions, cancers, diabetes mellitus. Non-communicable diseases have therefore taken a center stage and can no longer be ignored [7].

Studies have revealed that SSA carries one of the highest prostate cancer mortality rates in the world [8]. The Global Cancer (GLOBOCAN) 2012 noted an increased in the incidence and mortality rates of PCa for Africa which has reached 23.2 and 17.0 per 100,000 respectively [9]. In 2020, GLOBOCAN released another report which indicated that the incidence and mortality rate of PCa in Africa were 36.8 and 18.3 per 100,000, respectively. High incidences were found in Southern Africa with 65.1 per 100,000, followed by central Africa which had mortality rate of 24.8 per 10,000 and the lowest in North Africa with 16.6 per 10,000 men [9]. PCa was considered the second most diagnosed cancer in SSA and the fifth in mortality rates. Men in SSA suffer from PCA disproportionally as compared to men in other continents. The variations are attributed to genetic differences, dietary habits, poverty levels and presence of infectious diseases [10]. SSA, has for many decades been hit by the evolving and evolving communicable pandemics such as malaria, Ebola, AIDS and the recent COVID-19. The health focus has mainly been on these pandemics, with a lot of attention and resources being channeled into their management, care and prevention [11]. As a result, cancer care seems to have been disregarded despite the medical and social challenges it poses.

Tremendous strides have been made in the recent past improve people's lives globally and even in SSA. This has resulted in increased life expectancy of the population. However, as the population grows and life expectancy increases, there is an exponential increase in the cases of prostate cancer (PCa) [12]. Cancers cases, particularly the PCa have increased tremendously across SSA [13]. High incidences of PCA have been noticed in SSA and they seem to be growing at an alarming rate compared to other region in the world where incidence rates of PCa rates in most developed countries have stabilized and declining in others since 2012 [14]. However, within the SSA,

PCa has also been reported to be more common compared to other malignancy and constitute worse oncologic outcome. PCa in SSA has therefore become a major health concern in recent years and has the highest age standardized incidence and mortality rates of all cancers in men [15]. The 2020 GLOBOCAN program data revealed that it is the second most diagnosed cancer and is the fifth highest in mortality among men in the region [14].

A study conducted in 2021 to determine the rising prostate cancer incidence in sub-Saharan Africa revealed that rates of PCa have been increasing annually at the rate of 2–10% during the past decade [16] and predictions through demographic changes estimate that the number of incidences of prostate cancer will be more than double in SSA by 2030 [17]. This increase in the number of PCA cases will put more pressure on the healthcare systems in the region which are already struggling to manage the existing burden of cancers. While the healthcare systems are not yet robust to deal with the cancer problems, the situation is exacerbated by personal factors such as perceptions, culture and men's late response to the signs and symptoms and delayed diagnosis [18].

Incidence rates of prostate cancer vary substantially across the regions. The reason for the disparity is unclear but could be attributed to data management, access to medical care, screening practices and lifestyle factors among the population. A study done in 2021 reported a different demographic profile indicating that Southern Africa had its prevalence rates increased by 60%, while the highest mortality rates were realized in Western and Central regions [1].

In the past, PCa was commonly known to affect men in their advanced age. The landscape in SSA seems to be changing since more aggressive PCa is now being diagnosed among young men compared to developed countries even if the diagnosis is made at an advanced age [2]. Many men in the region normally present with more advance stages of the disease resulting in high mortality rates [3].

3. Care and management of PCa in sub Saharan Africa

The International Agency for Research on Cancer (IARC) GLOBOCAN program reported that prostate cancer (PCa) has become a serious medical and social problem in the world, but sub-Saharan Africa is experiencing the worst of its burden. The greatest concern for the condition comes with its diagnosis, management and secondary and tertiary care.

Globally, the commonest screening method for PCa involves using the prostate specific antigen (PSA) test. The test helps to detect the prostate cancer in the blood early and has been available for years. PSA is a protein produced only by the prostate and its high levels in the blood can indicate whether one has a cancer or not, however its elevation in the blood can also be caused by other common non-cancer related conditions such as an enlarged prostate—also known as benign prostatic hyperplasia or BPH, or prostatitis due to an infection or other cause. There is therefore some debate that arise from the benefits of using this test in men who show no signs of cancer. The reason for the controversy is that it does not yet meet the generally accepted criteria for a screening test. There is doubt on relying on it for diagnosis and treatment as well as screening which has led to some organization not to recommend its routine use particularly for screening.

Despite having been used for a long time and the controversies attached to its use, it remains the primary test for the PCa. Many countries in SSA do not always have this test, partly due to lack or have very few trained healthcare personnel to use it. In some other settings in SSA, the PSA test maybe be seen as an expensive screening method. The costs related to diagnosing and treating PCa primarily arise from accompanying test to conclude on the diagnosis and follow up investigations once the PSA is elevated. Some oncologists would prefer to confirm the presence of PCa and assess its stage and aggressiveness by performing other diagnostic procedures like biopsies and imaging scans. Doing these tests contribute to overall expenses that may be incurred by the patient. In SSA where medical care is medical expenses is not subsidized and it is out of the pocket, these tests are too expensive for an individual.

Physicians in SSA have stepped up in devising other test that can be recognized for early detection of PCa in SSA. The idea is to implement effective screening strategies that can consider age, family history, ethnicity, and other risk factors to identify individuals who are most likely to benefit from screening. There is another approach that has been developed and it uses alternative screening tools that are more accessible and affordable and is cost effective for SSA. In this approach, PSA levels that do not rely on laboratory quality control constraints is measured. The test is quick, simple, and similar to those used for rapid COVID-19 antigen tests. The test is at currently not commercially available, but when combined with digital rectal examination (DRE) it has proven to enhance access to PSA testing in settings with limited resources and financial constraints [7].

PCa in SSA is often diagnosed at an advanced stage due to the lack of access to screening and diagnostic facilities. The delay or lack of access to screening and diagnostic facilities often result in a poor prognosis and high mortality [8]. Many patients are not able to access a complete range of options in some parts of Africa and many men are not diagnosed at an early stage.

Since PSA testing and other diagnostic equipment are a challenge in SSA, physicians rely mainly on clinical evaluation and DRE to diagnose PCa. In some setting with better equipment, diagnosis is made based on clinical evaluation, DRE, MRI, biopsy, plain X-rays, and CT scans are also used in SSA. Nonetheless, access to these diagnostic measures is in many occasions limited, and expensive and not always available. As a result, some men in SSA may not receive an accurate diagnosis until the cancer has progressed to an advanced stage [9]. In some cancer centers, coming to a conclusive diagnosis takes some time. The patient may have to visit the health facility several times or even multiple healthcare providers before receiving a definitive diagnosis. These delay results in late diagnosis and late presentation of cancer at advanced stage. This challenge is compounded by the already disease burdened health facilities in SSA which are battling with HIV/AIDS, Acute respiratory tract conditions, tuberculosis, and malaria [19].

There is also variation in the screening across SSA. In East Africa for example, screening is less widely done when compared to West and Southern Africa. West and East Africa do not always do routine screening as part of medical care as it is the case in some settings in Southern Africa. Generally, most settings in SSA would do screening if a man presents with urinary symptoms and is over 50 years of age than those who are younger. South and West Africa are keen to screen men if they have a family history of PCa but this is not the case in East Africa [10].

An ultrasound guided biopsy of the prostate (TRUS) is commonly used in selected settings in South Africa to obtain a histopathological diagnosis of PCa. The method has been used in urological practice for over three decades. It has been refined to improve the detection rate of malignancy and has assisted in medical care of many patients.

It is performed under local anesthesia. It is however associated with some side effects such as pain, acute urinary retention, hematuria, hematospermia, rectal bleeding, erectile dysfunction, infection, and sepsis [11].

The option for treatment of PCa patients in SSA is always limited due to lack of resources such as access to diagnostic and treatment facilities, and a shortage of trained healthcare professionals. A study was conducted in 2022 to elicit insights into practices, norms, and values of PCa disparities and management in Southern Africa. The study revealed that there are inadequately available cancer care resources in Africa, including those used to manage PCa. The Oncologists are often faced with managing a broad spectrum of cancers. It was reported that oncologists, including those managing PCa in Africa have a significantly greater amount of clinical work and lower job satisfaction than their counterparts in various parts of the world. It has been assumed that the job dissatisfaction could be mainly due to limited medical devices and a lower doctor: patient ratio. For instance, African oncologists are estimated to be having a median number of 325 consults per year versus 175 of their counterparts in developed countries [12].

Insufficient professional healthcare providers has led to PCa screenings being performed by both trained medical personnel and in some cases by non-clinicians outside the medical system. It has been reported that there are variations in the reports by the trained personnel and the non-clinicians. This can jeopardize patients' outcomes and the significance of early diagnosis and timely access to treatment to optimize the patient's outcome [13]. However, available options include:

1. Surgery: Prostate surgery, (Prostatectomy) is the surgical removal of the prostate gland. The procedure is expensive and can only be instituted by the oncology or urology surgeon who can perform this complex surgery [12].

2. Radiation therapy: Due to shortages of the necessary high-quality equipment and clinical expertise, the treatment is limited. There is also need for repeated treatments requiring frequent visit to the health facility, or sometimes temporary relocation to get closer to the treatment center, or leave from work, all of which may be out of reach for many patients [8].

3. Androgen-deprivation therapy (ADT): This is a hormone therapy given primarily to help suppress prostate activity. The treatment is usually given to patient who have already progressed to an advanced stage at presentation and are often metastatic. This is in most instances combined with chemotherapy [14].

Due to disparity and poor access to healthcare services, many countries in Africa adopted the World Health Organization (WHO) initiative of palliative care as an additional key principle for effective cancer control in Low- and Middle-Income Countries (LMICs). The initiative aims to prevent or relief most suffering from serious or life-threatening health conditions and it can be taught easily to generalist clinicians who help and guide the care to be provided in the community. It requires only simple, inexpensive medicines and equipment [20]. Palliative care has been found to be the most appropriate strategy for PCa since most patients present at an advanced stage in radiotherapy and oncology centers, requiring the use of palliative radiotherapy, chemotherapy, hormonal care, analgesics, psychological and spiritual support [21].

4. Challenges in managing PCa in SSA

It has been well-documented that SSA is faced with increasing cases of PCa, SSA is also known to be faced with low economy which has impacted on the quality of infrastructure and healthcare delivery services. However, the statement cannot be applied to all countries in SSA. There are those which are in the Middle Income status and do have relatively good economy and healthcare services such as South Africa and Nigeria. Nonetheless, even in such countries there are still some disparities that affect access to PCa care. These disparities have led to numerous challenges relating to what the authors regard as two main categories, that is system and socio-economic factors.

4.1 Socio-economic factors

SSA mostly comprises of Low-Income Countries. Studies have shown that income improves the quality of health of the people, and there is a correlation between income and health. Higher income countries may have better healthcare infrastructures for its nationals, whereas people with low income may not be able to access good services and hence be confronted with stressful situations which are detrimental to their health [22].

The low level of economy does not only affect health but can be a determinant to large spheres of life. When there is not enough finance, pursuing education at an advanced level can be a problem and may lead to two main problems.

1. Lack of knowledge and inability to critique issues rationally, as well as poor drive to seek information. Education plays a major role in imparting knowledge to people and improving their perception and while on the other side, low literacy further hinders one to conceptualize basic instruction [23] and this may affect the way people perceive information on PCa. Studies have indicated that men with formal education are likely to comprehensively perceive messages about PCa and go for check-ups than their counterparts who do not have formal education [24, 25]. Conversely, people with low education or low literacy level have more perceived barriers. People with low literacy are not always keen to read and they would not understand instructions even when written in simplest terms.

2. Doubt, skepticism and mistrust are the core foundations for failure to change behavior and perception toward a condition even if its deadly. Knowledge is the judgment that is based on the ground that the judger recognizes to guarantees the truth of his judgment [26]. Some men in SSA are difficult to change their beliefs, perceptions and attitudes about PCa irrespective of how it causes suffering to them because of the prior knowledge and culture they hold [27]. Men in SSA are clouded with beliefs and attitudes that knowing about PCa cannot prevent them from having it, some belief it's one of the sexually transmitted infections while other hold fatalistic view that if they were destined to have PCa, nothing can stop it [28].

Africans are still holding on to their traditional cultural norms which may sometime be detrimental to their health. Some SSA men understand PCa as a contributing factor to erectile dysfunction even when their health is deteriorating and will reject the treatment or delay seeking medical help based on this belief. There are also beliefs associating PCa with a punishment from God, and that PCa is a curse because someone would have had sex with women of loose morals who infected him with bad blood and dirt that accumulates in their bodies. There have been personal views that not having enough sex leads to accumulation of spermatozoa in the body and hence leading to prostate cancer [29]. For an African man manhood and sexuality are important and integral part of their survival and always guard their sexuality jealously. All these beliefs and attitudes make men to respond poorly to their health care need, delay timely presentation for PCa care and present poor adherence to care and management.

Men have poor seeking behaviors and this does not change with generations. Men generally are perceived as leaders and heads in the family. The belief is that they must be strong and should never be seen as feeble nor visiting clinics or hospitals rather they should focus on working for the family. Men are to be physically, emotionally, socially and financially healthy and must be protectors of their families, ensuring stability within the household. A study conducted in South Africa unearth perceived traits of a strong man as someone drinking excessively, using drugs and practicing unprotected sex, all which are known to predispose to cancer [29].

It has been noted that managing prostate cancer requires a range of tests and procedures which are not common in SSA, and if available, will be expensive for out of hands payment by individuals. The larger part the SSA people are not working and cannot afford medical insurances. Therefore, they depend on government hospitals and clinics which are less expensive.

4.2 Healthcare system factors

Majority of the SSA men use the government health care systems. To access the health care, the patient has to go through the system which is multi-layered. Firstly, one has to go to the lowest level within the system being the clinic, which in most cases do not have specialist health care providers like physicians and oncologists. The next level is the district or county referral hospitals which may or sometime might not be having specialist. The last level is regional or national hospitals which have got specialist oncologist. This bureaucracy creates delays in which eventually the patient presents late to the oncologists. This kind of arrangement is available in Botswana, South Africa, Nigeria and other countries in SSA [30].

It has been documented that there is shortage of staff in the lower and medium level setting of the healthcare. An oncologist is appropriate personnel to diagnose and initiate a PCa on advanced treatment option. These specialists are only available in the higher echelon of the government healthcare system. A number of patients are sometimes lost along the way of this bureaucracy, some patients succumb to the condition during the delay while others complicate and the time they are seen by oncologist they are already in advanced stage of the disease.

Because of the centralist oncology care to tertiary or national hospitals, patients from rural areas, where the majority live incur a lot of expenses in accessing the services of these specialists. Furthermore, when a patient is hospitalized, the relatives willing to visit and give psychological support to him also incur a lot of costs as they have to find where to lodge or make repetitive visits to the hospital. In some cases, the relative would come sparingly leading to the patient feeling emotional low [29].

5. Conclusions

PCa among SSA men has been described as being aggressive at presentation with poor prognosis. This has been attributed to late presentation by the patients. The authors could not find any study that explains the reasons for the delayed presentation by PCa patients, but this has been associated with three main reasons. Firstly, men are generally poor in seeking medical help and therefore would delay until the situation is worsening. Additionally, men have got certain beliefs that hinder them from spontaneous respond to their conditions. These include, but not limited to masculinity belief, that they are strong and cannot easily complain, they belief PCa is one of the sexually transmitted infections and would first consult the traditional doctors before seeking modern medicine, they prioritize other chaos over seeking medical help, and they dislike the tests and examinations that are done to diagnose PCa. Lastly, the health care system has its own barriers. It is mainly multilayered, and this delays the referral flow, the lowest level which is a point of contact for PCa patients is mainly manned by females, particularly nurses. African men do not belief their genitalia have to be handled, especially by females. They equate this with insults and hence always delay because they do not want to be examined for PCa. The system also lacks enough qualified professional and therefore the doctor-patient ratio is too low, putting pressure on both the oncologists and the patients.

There is need for health care providers to increase awareness about PCa among the societies. Not only men, but everyone because PCa is a social problem and importantly when a man falls sick, he will ultimately be nursed by the entire family. Governments of different SSA region should devise *mind-set change* programs among men to appreciate the messages about PCa and the importance of testing. The programs should be tailored around the culture of every nation so that acceptance can be high.

Since the economies may not allow training, many oncologists and building structures should create space for PCa care in the rural areas, a deliberate effort can be made to train generalists and nurses on performing and initiating basic protocols for PCa care. An effort should also be made to modify cultures to accommodate that a man is a human being and mortal and conditions like PCa can affect him. Governments should strive to provide basic and not so expensive resources such as laboratory for PSA, clinical Psychologists, and prioritize PCa patients in the referral system. Strengthening the palliative care program and provision of incentives for men is important.

There is also a need for a robust study that will explore reasons for the late presentation by the PCa patients, experiences of PCa patients and their caretakers, and how to break through culture to facilitate uptake of PCa messages. Additionally, SSA governments must enforce register keeping for easy keeping of statistics.

Acknowledgements

The authors would like to sincerely thank the project Coordinator, Ms. Iva Horvat for the support and the confidence she showed in our determination and the commitment to complete the project, given our time limitations.

We also would like to extend our most sincere gratitude to the Librarian at the University of Botswana: Mr. T.W. Kophuting whose support in identifying articles and formatting the references, was unsurpassed.

Our most sincere appreciation also for the opportunity to work with such outstanding team of researchers. We do hope and wish there will be another opportunity for a continued partnership. We learned a lot during this collaboration.

Author's contributions

Both authors contributed to the completion of this manuscript. Their contribution is as follows: D. M. was responsible for concept formulation and formatting countercheck. W.M. B. took part in concept refinement, formatting and finalization. T.W. K., D. M., and W.M. B. conducted literature search. D.M. and W.M. B. extracted literature data and wrote the script.

Notes/thanks/other declarations

The authors would like to highly appreciate the management of IntechOpen for providing the template that is so user friendly. The authors did not struggle in settings up the manuscript, even the instructions provided are easy to understand and follow.

Acronyms and abbreviations

ADT	androgen deprivation therapy
AIDS	acquired immune deficiency syndrome
CT scan	computed tomography
DRE	digital rectal examination
GLOBOCAN	Global Cancer
HIV	human immune-deficiency virus
LMICs	Low- and Middle-Income Countries
MRI	magnetic resonance imaging
PCa	prostate cancer
PSA	prostate-specific antigen
SSA	sub-Saharan Africa
TRUSS	the transrectal ultrasound scan
WHO	World Health Organization

Author details

Ditsapelo M. McFarland[1*] and William M. Baratedi[2]

1 College of Nursing and Public Health, Adelphi University, Garden City, NY, USA

2 School of Nursing, University of Botswana, Gaborone, Botswana

*Address all correspondence to: dmcfarland@adelphi.edu

IntechOpen

© 2024 The Author(s). Licensee IntechOpen. This chapter is distributed under the terms of the Creative Commons Attribution License (http://creativecommons.org/licenses/by/4.0), which permits unrestricted use, distribution, and reproduction in any medium, provided the original work is properly cited.

References

[1] Ngoran SD, Xue XZ, Wesseh PK Jr. Signatures of water resources consumption on sustainable economic growth in sub-Saharan African countries. International Journal of Sustainable Built Environment. 2016;**5**(1):114-122

[2] Gasparatos A et al. Sustainability challenges in sub-Saharan Africa: Trade-offs, opportunities and priority areas for sustainability science. In: Sustainability Challenges in Sub-Saharan Africa II: Insights from Eastern and Southern Africa. Singapore Pte Ltd; 2020. pp. 245-262

[3] Food and Agriculture Organization of the United Nations. The Future of Food and Agriculture: Trends and Challenges. Rome: FAO; 2017

[4] United Nations, Department of Economic and Social Affairs, Population Division. World population prospects: The 2017 revision, key findings and advance tables. In: Working Paper No. ESA/P/WP/248. New York: United Nations; 2017. p. 46

[5] World Bank. The World Bank Annual Report 2017, 2017. Washington DC: The World Bank;

[6] WHO Regional Office for Africa. Communicable and Non-communicable Diseases in Africa 2021/22. Brazzaville: World Health Organization; 2023

[7] Gouda HN et al. Burden of non-communicable diseases in sub-Saharan Africa, 1990-2017: Results from the Global Burden of Disease Study 2017. The Lancet Global Health. 2019;**7**(10):e1375-e1387

[8] Bray F et al. Global cancer statistics 2018: GLOBOCAN estimates of incidence and mortality worldwide for 36 cancers in 185 countries. CA: A Cancer Journal for Clinicians. 2018;**68**(6):394-424

[9] Sung H et al. Global cancer statistics 2020: GLOBOCAN estimates of incidence and mortality worldwide for 36 cancers in 185 countries. CA: A Cancer Journal for Clinicians. 2021;**71**(3):209-249

[10] Adeloye D et al. An estimate of the incidence of prostate cancer in Africa: A systematic review and meta-analysis. PLoS ONE. 2016;**11**(4):e0153496

[11] Parkin DM, Ferlay J, Jemal A. et al. Cancer in Sub-Saharan Africa. International Agency for Research on Cancer. France: IARC Scientific Publications – No. 167. WHO; 2018. ISBN 978-92-832-2221-7. ISSN 0300-5085

[12] Culp MB et al. Recent global patterns in prostate cancer incidence and mortality rates. European Urology. 2020;**77**(1):38-52

[13] Andrews C et al. Development, evaluation, and implementation of a pan-African cancer research network: Men of African descent and carcinoma of the prostate. Journal of Global Oncology. 2018;**4**:1-14

[14] Ferlay J et al. Global cancer observatory. Cancer Today. 2018;**23**(7):323-326

[15] Seraphin TP et al. Rising prostate cancer incidence in sub-Saharan Africa: A trend analysis of data from the African cancer registry network. Cancer Epidemiology, Biomarkers & Prevention. 2021;**30**(1):158-165

[16] Cassell A et al. A review of localized prostate cancer: An African perspective. World Journal of Oncology. 2019;**10**(4-5):162

[17] Chu LW et al. Prostate cancer incidence rates in Africa. Prostate Cancer. 2011;**2011**(1):947870

[18] Hamdi Y et al. Cancer in Africa: The untold story. Frontiers in Oncology. 2021;**11**:650117

[19] Rebbeck TR et al. Global patterns of prostate cancer incidence, aggressiveness, and mortality in men of African descent. Prostate Cancer. 2013;**2013**(1):560857

[20] Planning WHO. Implementing Palliative Care Services: A Guide for Programme Managers. Geneva: World Health Organization. WHO Library Cataloguing-in-publication Data; 2016

[21] Adamu A et al. Outcomes in palliative care for advanced prostate cancer in the radiotherapy and oncology department of the Ahmadu Bello university teaching hospital, Zaria. Nigerian Journal of Medicine. 2018;**27**(1):1-6

[22] Lenhart O. The effects of income on health: New evidence from the Earned Income Tax Credit. Review of Economics of the Household. 2019;**17**(2):377-410

[23] Roberts A. Barriers Preventing Early Detection of Prostate cancer in Black African/Caribbean Men Living in Westminster. Westminster: Westminister's Jointy Strategic Needs Assessment; 2010

[24] Ojewola RW et al. Knowledge, attitudes and screening practices regarding prostatic diseases among men older than 40 years: A population-based study in Southwest Nigeria. The Pan African Medical Journal. 30 Jun 2017;**27**:151. pp. 1-6. DOI: 10.11604/pamj.2017.27.151.10605. PMID: 28904679; PMCID: PMC5567951

[25] Wanyagah P. Prostate cancer awareness, knowledge, perception on self-vulnerability and uptake of screening among men in Nairobi County, Kenya. Kenyatta University Institutional Repository. 2014;**2014**:92

[26] Kern A. Kant on doubt and error. Midwest Studies in Philosophy. 2021;**45**:129-154

[27] Marima R et al. Prostate cancer disparities and management in southern Africa: Insights into practices, norms and values. Cancer Management and Research. 2022;**14**:3567-3579. DOI: 10.2147/CMAR.S382903

[28] Baratedi WM et al. Barriers to prostate cancer screening by men in sub-Saharan Africa: An integrated review. Journal of Nursing Scholarship. 2020;**52**(1):85-94

[29] Nzama N. Masculinity and Men's Health Seeking Behaviours amongst Black/African Men: The Case of Durban, KwaZulu-Natal, South Africa. Durban, South Africa: University of KwaZulu Natal; 2013

[30] Koce F, Randhawa G, Ochieng B. Understanding healthcare self-referral in Nigeria from the service users' perspective: A qualitative study of Niger state. BMC Health Services Research. 2019;**19**:1-14